THE

Migraine
Relief Plan

COOKBOOK

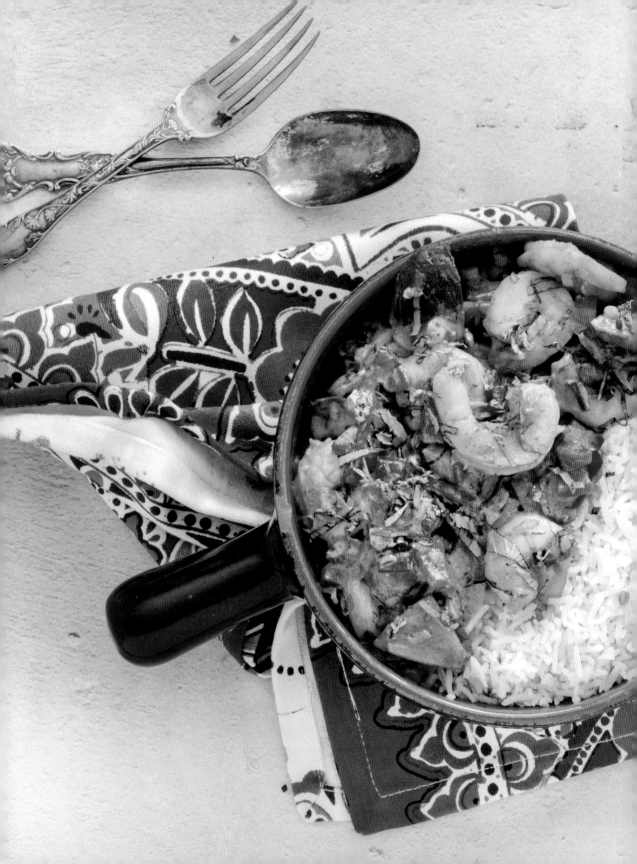

THE
Migraine
Relief Plan
COOKBOOK

More Than 100 Anti-Inflammatory
Recipes for Managing Headaches and
Living a Healthier Life

Stephanie Weaver, MPH

SURREY
BOOKS

AN AGATE IMPRINT

CHICAGO

This book is intended to supplement, not replace, the advice of a trained
health professional. If you know or suspect that you have a health problem,
you should consult with a health professional. The author and publisher
specifically disclaim any liability, loss, or risk, personal or otherwise, that is
incurred as a consequence, directly or indirectly, of the use and application
of any of the contents of this book.

The field of migraine medicine and research is always changing.
This book reflects the state of knowledge when it went to publication.

First printed in July 2022

Printed in China

10 9 8 7 6 5 4 3 2 1   22 23 24 25 26

Cataloging-in-Publication Data is available from the Library of Congress.

ISBN 13: 978-1-57284-311-0
ISBN 10: 1-57284-311-X
eISBN 13: 978-1-57284-859-7
eISBN 10: 1-57284-859-6

Surrey Books is an imprint of Agate Publishing. Agate books are available
in bulk at discount prices. For more information, visit agatepublishing.com.

For everyone living with chronic illness, including my friends in the migraine community.

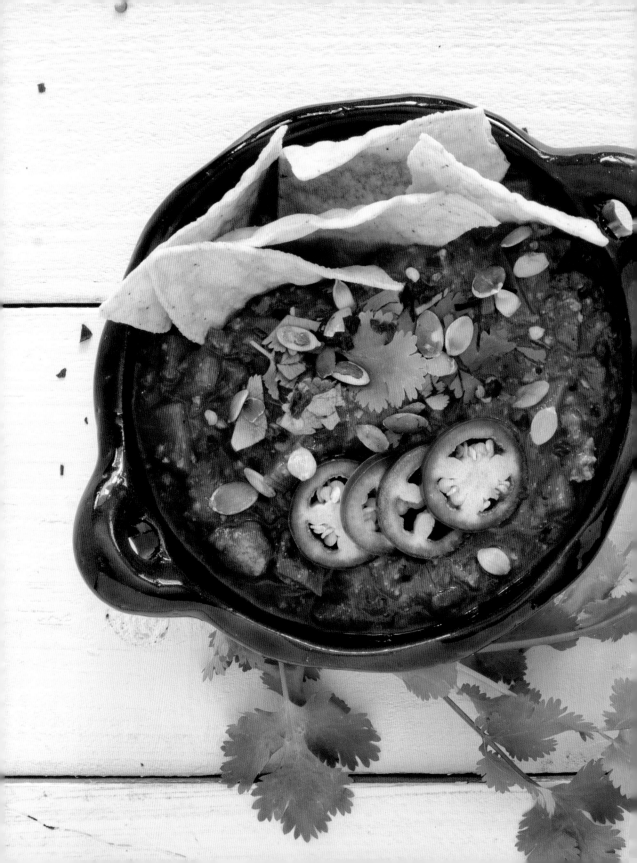

Contents

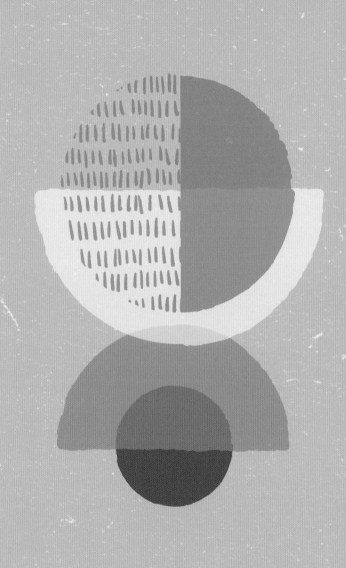

Foreword

RESILIENCE IS DEFINED AS an ability to recover from or adjust to challenges or change. Or, as meditation researcher Jon Kabat-Zinn put it, "You can't stop the waves, but you can learn to surf." Living with any chronic disease is a series of adjusting to challenges. Resilience is how we "surf." Living with migraine disease can be challenging. It's important to care for both body and mind by enhancing physical and psychological health and resilience. While there is currently no cure for migraine, there are a wide range of actions and treatments that play a major role in managing migraine attacks, enhancing resilience, and allowing you to live the life that you want to live. The goals of migraine management are to prevent attacks when possible, and to shorten the intensity, duration, and disability of those that do occur, using non-medication and medication approaches. Eating well is one of the foundational lifestyle aspects that can enhance physical and psychological resilience.

Migraine is a common disease that is estimated to affect more than 1 billion people around the world and an estimated 40 million Americans.[1,2,3] Migraine has been with humans since the beginning of recorded human history! Fortunately, our scientific understanding of migraine is constantly evolving, and we have recently learned a great deal. Migraine has a genetic predisposition, meaning that it runs in families, and the risk of having migraine is carried in your DNA. Migraine is not your fault. As a chronic disease with episodic manifestations, someone with migraine always has the disease, but migraine attacks may occur on an unpredictable basis.[4] We refer to headache and other symptoms such as nausea, sensitivity to light and sound, fatigue, and feeling fuzzy-headed as a migraine attack. A migraine attack can last several days, has several phases, and has many symptoms in addition to headache. (For more information about migraine, including information about diagnosis, attack phases, and symptoms, see page 6).

Someone with migraine has a sensitive nervous system that responds to changes in the internal and external environment. These risk factors are often called "triggers." A migraine attack can happen when the combination of biological and environmental risk factors exceeds an individual's biological threshold. Some people can sense when a migraine attack is about to happen and feel that certain situations and/or events might make an attack more likely. Other people feel that attacks happen out of the blue. Risk factors can stack up to raise the risk of an attack, and if they pass over a biological migraine attack threshold, an attack may occur. Everyone has a migraine attack threshold, which can rise or lower depending on a variety of external and internal variables. Some ways to raise this threshold to reduce the chance of migraine attacks and stack the odds in your favor include healthy nutrition, regular exercise or movement, managing stress, and other healthy habits. When attempting to prevent migraine attacks through lifestyle, it can be helpful to think of a two-pronged approach: raising the threshold and lowering risk factors and triggers.

> When attempting to prevent migraine attacks through lifestyle, it can be helpful to think of a two-pronged approach: **raising the threshold and lowering risk factors and triggers.**

The most common risk factors or triggers are related to changes in routines. For some people, risk factors or triggers can include skipping meals, dehydration, stress, relaxation after a stressful period, too much or too little sleep, changing sleep patterns, and weather changes. Some people notice they are more likely to have a migraine attack after eating or drinking certain foods. Research shows that changes in routines like varying the amount of caffeine a person drinks from day to day can be a risk factor. In many women, monthly hormonal changes can be risk factors as well. A combination of lowered threshold combined with risk factors may set the stage for a migraine attack. For example, college students may feel stress studying for finals week. They may not get enough sleep, skip some meals, grab fast food, drink extra coffee, and end up having a migraine attack on the first day of spring break. This does not mean they caused the migraine attack (remember that migraine is a disease with a genetic predisposition). But whenever possible, we want to practice healthy lifestyle habits to try to buffer against the difficult challenges that happen in life. The nervous system of a person with migraine thrives with healthy habits and consistency.

Fortunately, there is a core set of healthy lifestyle habits which enhance our resilience and can be a big help in managing migraine, likely by regulating the nervous system and raising the threshold for attacks. These habits involve keeping a regular, healthy routine around eating, hydration, sleep, and exercise, plus managing stress and maximizing social support.

When it comes to nutrition, the current evidence for dietary approaches to managing migraine aligns in many ways with what is broadly accepted as healthy nutrition. While many divergent dietary patterns have been studied for their impact on migraine (low-carb, low-fat, ketogenic, and so forth), the diets with beneficial effects have significant overlap in the types of foods they provide. This includes an overall eating pattern that focuses on whole foods, provides large quantities of vegetables and sometimes fruits, chooses whole grains over refined grains whenever possible, limits sugars, and aims for proteins to come from lean sources, especially plant-based proteins and fatty, omega-3–rich fish. This eating pattern is consistent with dietary patterns that reduce inflammation in the body.[5] Lower inflammation resulting from diet may influence migraine and has already been shown to decrease risks associated with many other chronic diseases of inflammation that occur alongside migraine, such as heart disease, depression, anxiety, allergies, and obesity.[6] Recent evidence shows that other mechanisms may also be at play, including an anti-pain effect when omega-3 fat intake is increased in the diet, especially alongside decreases in omega-6 fats.[7]

> Whenever possible, we want to practice healthy lifestyle habits to try to buffer against the difficult challenges that happen in life.

Further nutritional actions like eating regularly to maintain steady blood sugar levels, drinking unsweetened beverages to stay hydrated, and achieving and maintaining a healthy weight are important for everyone's physical health, but these actions also take on extra importance in managing migraine.

What and when we eat and drink and when we sleep and exercise are areas we can control, yet it can be challenging to make these changes. We all know how difficult it can be both to start and to maintain healthy lifestyle changes. We may want to and know that we should, but life gets in the way. We may be in pain, too busy, too tired, not have enough time, money, or energy...and that's when motivation becomes so important. Having delicious, nutritious recipes to try like those in this book can help motivate us on the path to making a healthy habit change. It may be heartening to hear that exercise, diet, and sleep routines also work together in the body to support each other and make it easier for you to maintain the changes over time. For example, regular exercise has been shown to control appetite, and a nutritional, quality diet is associated with better sleep. The combination of these healthy habits keeps our bodies healthy, balanced, and resilient.

When it comes to sleep, it is important to get enough restorative sleep and also to try to go to bed and wake up at about the same time every day. For exercise, it's encouraged to engage in exercise or movement on most days. In addition, stress management, participating in enjoyable and relaxing activities, and social support also help us live well with migraine. Living with migraine can take its toll both physically and emotionally. And while we cannot always control the things that happen to us, practicing stress management (how we react to things) and relaxation techniques can help raise our migraine threshold and make attacks less likely. Many people practice stress management and relaxation on their own or with self-guided approaches, while some work with professionals to learn the scientifically proven behavioral migraine management techniques: biofeedback, cognitive behavioral therapy, relaxation therapies, mindfulness-based therapies, and acceptance and commitment therapy.[8] It's important to note that if stress, depression, or anxiety feel unmanageable, you can talk to your doctor or a mental healthcare provider. In addition, half of all people living with migraine have not been diagnosed or talked to a healthcare professional about it. There are many treatment options available when working with a healthcare professional. If you experience migraine or other headaches that are disabling or interfere with your life, consider talking with your healthcare professional to receive a medical diagnosis and discuss a personalized treatment plan for you, which may include non-medication and medication options.

When it comes to managing migraine, consistency is key. Practicing healthy habits on a consistent basis will also strengthen resilience and improve physical and mental well-being. Migraine is a chronic disease with unpredictable, painful, and potentially debilitating attacks that can take a toll both physically and emotionally, but there are many healthy habits that are key to successful migraine management. These habits increase resilience and help you stay physically and psychologically healthy. It is essential to raise the migraine attack threshold with healthy habits, including eating well, being aware of and managing triggers and risk factors, and maintaining a healthy lifestyle. Healthy and consistent routines for nutrition, hydration, sleep, exercise or movement, relaxation, and stress management enhance resilience and translate to benefits for the nervous system and therefore the whole person. These actions not only help reduce the frequency, impact, and burden of migraine attacks, but also translate into benefits for your entire well-being. The recipes and strategies in this book provide healthy, nutritious, and delicious food options to make both your body and your taste buds happy.

Be well,

Margaret Slavin, PhD, RDN
Dawn C. Buse, PhD

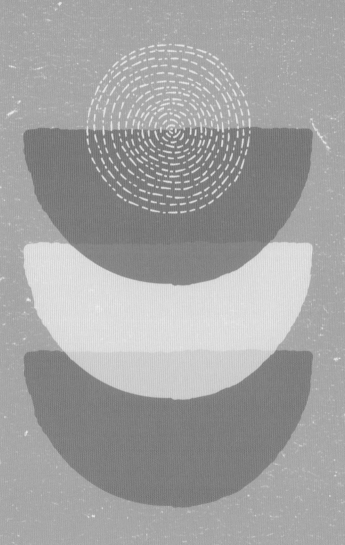

Introduction

Why I wrote this cookbook for you

Hɪ, I'ᴍ Sᴛᴇᴘʜᴀɴɪᴇ. At the age of fifty-three, after a few bouts of severe vertigo and a lifetime of what I thought of as "weather headaches," I was diagnosed with vertigo with migraine variant—a diagnosis that would change my life. I knew very little about migraine disease at the time, or that lifestyle factors could affect how frequent or severe my attacks might be. I only knew that I was wicked dizzy, and I wanted the world to stop spinning. The two doctors I saw, an otolaryngologist (formerly called ear, nose, and throat doctors) and a neurologist specializing in balance disorders, each gave me a prescription. Most importantly, each gave me a handout with dietary recommendations. One sheet covered low-sodium diets; the other introduced me to a version of the migraine diet restricting foods containing something called tyramine, a naturally occurring compound found in aged and fermented foods, among others. But that was it; those handouts had extremely limited information.

With my background as a recipe developer, food blogger, and health-and-wellness coach, and with a master's in public health in nutrition education, focusing on food as a way to deal with my diagnosis made sense to me. As I began to feel better, it bothered me that there was so little out there to help other people. Not only did I have that degree in public health, I'd been "renovating" recipes my entire adult life—taking traditional recipes and adjusting them for special diets—and had been writing a food blog called *Recipe Renovator* for three years. (It's now MigraineReliefRecipes.com.) In my previous work in museum education I'd become well versed in curriculum development. Maybe *I* was the one who needed to write the book I'd needed. Thus began my journey into Migraine-Diet-Land, setting the stage for me to develop the eight-week approach I detail in *The*

1

Migraine Relief Plan (Surrey Books, 2017) and ultimately the recipes in this follow-up cookbook.

I had wanted *The Migraine Relief Plan* to make readers feel like they had a migraine-wellness coach by their side, helping them gradually adjust their habits over a period of months to incorporate regular movement, sleep, hydration, and a meditation or relaxation practice. As I shared information online about migraine disease and attended conferences and patient-education days at headache centers, I met some amazing migraine advocates and physicians who inspired me and informed this book, including Dr. Dawn Buse and Dr. Margaret Slavin, who co-wrote the Foreword. As I became more involved with online communities and began to identify myself as someone with chronic illnesses (migraine disease, fibromyalgia, and thyroid disease), I met more friends and saw the continued value in speaking out and sharing resources like the Migraine World Summit annual online conference, the Miles for Migraine run/walk events around the US, and the annual RetreatMigraine patient conference. I watched as my community on Facebook helped each other, answered questions, and shared their own Plan-friendly recipes. I invite you to join us; just search "migraine relief plan" on Facebook.

Before I started to work on the recipes for this book, I issued a survey to my readers. They told me they needed *more snacks*. They also wanted more breakfast ideas and light meals for migraine-attack days. They wanted to do more bulk cooking on the weekends, to know what to do with leftovers, to have more vegetarian options, and they asked for "fewer fish recipes." This last one made me laugh, because out of seventy-five recipes in the first book only five include fish or seafood. (A recent study provides encouraging evidence that eating fatty fish and reducing seed oils, such as soybean and canola, may help reduce the severity and frequency of attacks.[9]) Readers also wanted recipes that were simpler, so I worked to streamline the ingredients and steps in the ones you'll find here. They will still turn out beautifully and tempt the taste buds of everyone in the family.

Once I had the list of proposed recipes that met all those criteria, I prepared each one at least three times in my home kitchen, often sharing the results with neighbors for feedback. Once I was satisfied that a recipe was excellent, I sent it to my volunteer testing crew of over forty people in four countries. Each recipe was tested by at least three people to make sure the instructions were clear and the results were outstanding. I share this because I want you to trust that every recipe will turn out for you in your kitchen. I am so grateful to them for persevering through the challenges of the pandemic, despite limited grocery runs and ingredient shortages.

Finally, I sent the recipes to experts in Southeast Asian, Indian, Mexican, and Mediterranean cuisines to make sure they were culturally sensitive and appropriate. The most fun was watching the recipes come to life as my stellar food photographer, Laura Bashar of *Family Spice*, shot the images for this book.

The recipes are divided into the following chapters: Snacks, Breakfast, Salads and Light Meals, Weekend Cooking, Scrumptious Sides, Progressive Cooking (three base recipes, plus options to make dishes with the leftovers), Desserts, and Sauces, Condiments, and Basics.

One tester asked if I could include serving suggestions for each recipe, so you'll find those on each page, and there are menu collections for special occasions in the back.

In the Appendix you'll find the full recipe list with recipes coded as Vegetarian/Vegan, Dairy-Free, Egg-Free, and Grain-Free. (You'll find icons for those categories on the recipes themselves.)

After this introduction, you'll find an overview of the Plan, a two-page explanation of how the full Plan works, and a list of which foods to eliminate and which to include if you're following the elimination portion. Then come more than 115 new recipes, the heart of this cookbook.

The trigger controversy

The Migraine Relief Plan supports people in systematically shifting their eating for a few months to determine if they have recognizable food triggers. Once the testing period is completed, readers are encouraged to add back all foods that don't cause problems for them.

When I wrote *The Migraine Relief Plan*, I didn't know migraine diets were considered controversial, due to a lack of high-quality research. I have learned over the years that while food triggers are considered controversial, doctors agree that migraine is an inflammatory condition that may be moderated with an anti-inflammatory diet and lifestyle changes. While the parameters of anti-inflammatory diets differ, most feature a diet rich in whole foods, low in processed foods and sugars, and low in certain oils (the kind found in processed foods). All the recipes in this and my first book fit that description.

While it was frustrating to learn that some doctors considered my book controversial, two things have kept me going on this path. The first are the doctors who loved the book and recommended it to their migraine patients. I heard from my own neurologist that he was now putting all his patients on the Plan, even those without migraine disease, because the anti-inflammatory benefits were proving so helpful overall. Second are the messages and emails from readers who told me that my book changed their life. That they attended a son's or daughter's wedding and were able to enjoy it. That their migraine pattern was greatly improved. That they loved being able to cook for their partner with migraine disease knowing the foods they made could help them feel better.

While food triggers are considered controversial, doctors agree that migraine is an inflammatory condition that may be moderated with an anti-inflammatory diet and lifestyle changes.

Resilience

Living with a chronic condition like migraine disease is not easy. So in addition to providing beautiful, appealing recipes, I wanted this book to give readers ongoing inspiration. That got me thinking about the power of resilience.

Resilience is not something one has or doesn't. It is built through regular, sustained practice. Beginning in 2020, I conducted a series of interviews called *The Resilience Series*. I talked to patients and advocates with migraine and other chronic disease, migraine researchers and doctors, health professionals, and writers exploring stories of resilience. You'll find quotes from those interviews sprinkled throughout the recipe section. They're meant to inspire you, whether you're a patient, a provider, or a caregiver cooking for a loved one. You'll find the video interviews on Facebook, Instagram, and YouTube.

I am grateful to all the people who provided their time and expertise to create the book you're holding in your hands. It's not my book. It's our book.

Here's to leading a beautiful, resilient life, regardless of the challenges that come our way.

The Migraine Threshold Theory

Migraine disease is a neuro-biological condition with a hereditary component. While doctors don't agree about food triggers because the research has not been definitive, they do agree that there are attack triggers and that those triggers are cumulative.

In his book *The Migraine Miracle*, Dr. Josh Turknett uses the metaphor of a hot air balloon to illustrate the migraine threshold theory. Imagine that your life is a ride in your own personal hot air balloon. You need to stay below a dangerous height. Getting enough sleep and gentle movement, as well as staying hydrated, all help lower the balloon to a safe height. Eating whole foods that are anti-inflammatory lowers you. And, if you are among those of us who have food triggers, avoiding them lowers you further. If you are able to glide well below your unique threshold, you can weather a few of these triggers on any given day or week. But if you have a stressful week, eat convenience foods that don't fit your meal plan, have a cocktail, and get to bed late, the combination of these factors might raise you past your threshold. My Plan helps you identify your unique triggers and figure out what you can control so you can live as much as possible well below your personal threshold.

> My Plan helps you identify your unique triggers and figure out what you can control so you can live as much as possible well below your personal threshold.

What Is a Migraine Attack?

Headache is usually, but not always, the main symptom, and can last from 4 to 72 hours if untreated. The headache is often, but not necessarily, unilateral (one-sided), with pulsating pain, and aggravated by movement or activity. Migraine attacks also often involve nausea, vomiting, photophobia (sensitivity to light), phonophobia (sensitivity to sound), and osmophobia (sensitivity to smell), as well as other associated symptoms. There are also subtypes of migraine with additional symptoms such as vertigo. In addition to pain, these associated symptoms can make it very difficult to function. Many people prefer to rest in a dark and quiet place during the headache phase. If possible, it is often preferred to sleep or at least lie down. Sleep can be very restorative for the nervous system.

The prodrome is a phase that can occur from 12 to 24 hours preceding the actual headache. Symptoms may include irritability, neck pain or stiffness, food cravings, or yawning, in addition to other symptoms. The postdrome phase can occur 12 to 24 hours after the headache has resolved. Much like the prodrome, during this time someone may report not feeling like themselves, may have difficulty thinking clearly, and feel fatigued or washed out.

About one in five people experience aura with a migraine attack. An aura may last for 5 to 60 minutes before the headache begins and includes sensory changes. Most commonly, aura includes visual changes such as seeing flickering lights, spots, or lines, or losing a portion of the visual field. Other senses can also be involved. With a sensory aura a person may experience numbness, the sensation of pins and needles, or weakness. Aura can also affect the ability to speak, and can lead to confusion or dizziness. The experience of aura may change from attack to attack and they can be very distressing, especially the first time it happens.

In light of all four phases, a migraine attack can last for several days. It can incapacitate someone or limit their ability to function for an extended period of time. Migraine can negatively affect all aspects of life, including work, school, family, socializing, hobbies, mood, and well-being.[10] As a result, migraine can also negatively impact the lives of those close to us: family members, friends, coworkers, and community. In addition, it can be difficult to plan or make commitments due to uncertainty about when the next attack will occur.

The Migraine Relief Plan

Diet and The Migraine Relief Plan

The Migraine Relief Plan supports you in shifting eating habits for a few months to determine if you have recognizable food triggers, and it should help reduce inflammation in your body. Some percentage of people with migraine disease have recognizable food triggers. (Though as I write in the Introduction, this is controversial.) Possibly another slice of people has food sensitivities (which they might discover through specialized testing), which could add to their body's inflammatory response. But all people with migraine disease are likely to benefit from a whole foods, anti-inflammatory eating plan.

That's where the recipes in this book come in. You can use any of them while following the elimination portion of my Plan, or use them for general health and wellness, as they are all anti-inflammatory, gluten-free, nut-free (except for coconut), low in sodium, and nearly free of added sugar. The Plan is supportive of everyone, because it's built around anti-inflammatory foods. It may help address diabetes and other chronic conditions that often occur with migraine. Once the testing period is completed, add back whole foods that don't cause issues.

What follows is an overview of the Plan and a list of foods so you can see at a glance which to include and which to avoid if you're experimenting with the elimination diet phase of the Plan.

The Migraine Relief Plan Overview

- Eat whole foods, lots of vegetables, and healthy fats to help reduce inflammation and support your overall health.
- Develop a regular sleep and wake schedule.
- Drink plenty of water.
- Maintain a steady blood sugar level throughout the day.
- Incorporate gentle movement gradually, even if you can't work out.
- Build a meditation or relaxation practice into your day.
- Consider environmental triggers like lighting, scents, and sounds.

The full Plan involves devoting six or so months to experimenting with the elimination diet to determine if you have food triggers that may be unknown to you, or if certain common ingredients in the Standard American Diet (salt, sugar, low-quality oils, and wheat flour containing gluten) may be playing a role in your migraine pattern. If this doesn't feel possible for you, you can simply use the 115 recipes in this book, plus the 75 recipes in *The Migraine Relief Plan,* and see how you feel. But note that these recipes are free from a lot of healthful foods too, such as citrus, nuts, avocados, and many beans, so adding those foods back is optimal for the long-term if they are not triggers for you.

One final note: If you have struggled with disordered eating, please consult a dietitian or nutritionist who is knowledgeable about it and can guide you. It may be that tracking food and symptoms could cause your eating disorder to flare up, so proceed with caution. You can still follow the Plan by utilizing the many recipes in both books.

The Migraine Relief Plan

Week	Assignments	Daily Steps	Daily Active Minutes	Daily Sodium (mg)	Daily Caffeine (cups)	Daily Sugar
MONTH 1: Begin tracking; reduce salt and caffeine; slowly increase movement						
Week 1	Set up tracking system	Regular routine	Regular routine	Regular routine	Regular routine	Regular routine
Week 2	Freezer cleanout	4,000	5	3,000	2	
Week 3	Pantry cleanout	5,000	10 (2–3 days per week)	2,500	1½	
Week 4	Fridge cleanout Switch snacks to Plan	6,000	15 (2–3 days per week)	2,000	1	
MONTH 2: Switch meals to the Plan one week at a time; reduce then eliminate sugar						
Week 5	Switch breakfast to Plan	7,000	20 (2–3 days per week)	1,500	½	1 snack per day
Week 6	Switch lunch to Plan	8,000	25 (2–3 days per week)	1,200–1,500	0	1 snack per week
Week 7	Switch dinner to Plan	9,000	30 (2–3 days per week)	1,000–1,500		0
Week 8	Special order at restaurant	10,000		1,000–1,500		0
MONTH 3: Add self-care and mind/body activities						
Week 9 **Week 10** **Week 11** **Week 12**	• Make an appointment for bodywork • Buy or record a guided meditation and listen to it at least once • Try a priming exercise • Take 15 minutes to write about how you're feeling about having to give up your favorite foods; wallow and move on • Talk to a friend and ask for 1–2 things they can do to help you	10,000	30 (2–3 days per week)	1,000–1,500	0	0

Week	Assignments	Daily Steps	Daily Active Minutes	Daily Sodium (mg)	Daily Caffeine (cups)	Daily Sugar
MONTH 4: Detox your body and environment						
Week 13	• Try dry brushing	10,000	30 (2–3 days per week)	1,000–1,500	0	0
Week 14	• Go barefoot on the grass or at the beach					
Week 15	• Make 1 room in your home healthier for you					
Week 16	• Make 1 aspect of your work environment healthier for you					
MONTH 5: Planning to fail						
Week 17	• Restaurant recon	10,000	30 (2–3 days per week)	1,000–1,500	0	0
Week 18	• Plan 1 thing that will help you through the next holiday gathering					
Week 19	• Plan for an upcoming vacation					
Week 20	• Think of ways you can be more supportive of yourself if you were to "fail" on the Plan					
MONTH 6: Sleep and movement						
Week 21	• Make your bedroom a sleep haven	10,000	30 (2–3 days per week)	1,000–1,500	0	0
Week 22	• Try listening to white noise or a guided sleep meditation for a few nights					
Week 23	• Think about what you really love to do that's active rather than what you think you "should" do; plan those activities					
Week 24	• Focus on lots of little movements (not "working out")					
MONTH 7 AND ON: Start trigger testing and reintroducing foods						
Week 25	• Make your list of foods you want to test	10,000	30 (2–3 days per week)	1,000–1,500	0	0
Week 26	• Restart tracking if you have stopped for a while					
Week 27	• Follow the trigger testing guidelines and experiment					
Week 28						

The Migraine Relief Plan Food List

Grains

Approved	Amaranth Corn (tortillas, tortilla chips, polenta) Garbanzo bean (chickpea) flour Gluten-free bread (choose whole-grain and low-sodium where possible) Gluten-free pasta Millet Oats (certified gluten-free) Quinoa Rice Sorghum Tapioca (pearls and flour) Teff
Excluded	Wheat berries; couscous; cracked wheat; rye; barley; spelt; triticale; einkorn; farro; white, wheat, or all-purpose flour; garfava flour

Veggies and beans

Approved	Adzuki beans Artichokes Arugula Asparagus Bamboo shoots Beet greens Beets Bell peppers Bitter melon Bok choy Broccoli Brussels sprouts Cabbage Cactus leaves (nopales) Cardoni Carrots Cauliflower Celery Celery root Chickpeas Chile peppers Chives Cilantro Corn Cucumbers Daikon Eggplant Fennel Galangal root Garlic Gingerroot Green beans (haricot verts) Green onions (scallions, spring onions) Greens (such as mustard, dandelion, collard) Horseradish (fresh) Jerusalem artichokes (sunchokes) Jicama Kale Kidney beans Kohlrabi Leeks Lettuce Lotus root Mung beans Mushrooms Parsley Parsnips Peas Perilla Pinto beans Potatoes Pumpkins Radishes Rutabagas Salsify Shallots Spinach Split peas Squash (all, including summer squash and zucchini) Sweet potatoes Swiss chard Taro Tomatillos Tomatoes Truffles Turnips Wax beans White beans Yams Yucca
Excluded	Broad beans, fava beans, Italian beans, lentils, lima beans, navy beans, onions, pea pods, sauerkraut, snow pea pods
Notes	• Fresh sprouts are OK if from approved list. • Fresh vegetables on the list may be dried in a home dehydrator. • Home-canned sauces, made from fresh ingredients, are fine. • Dried chiles and mushrooms are OK without sulfites.

Fruits

Approved			
Apples	Dragon fruit	Mangoes	Purple plums
Apricots	Gooseberries	Mangosteens	Quince
Blackberries	Grapes	Melons (all)	Rambutans
Blueberries	Guavas	Nectarines	Rhubarb
Cactus pears (prickly pear fruit)	Jujubes (the fruit, not the candy)	Peaches	Sapotes
		Pears	Starfruit
Cherimoyas	Kiwis	Persimmons	Tamarind (without sugar or sulfites if dried/paste)
Cherries	Longans	Plumcots	
Coconuts	Loquats	Pluots	
Cranberries	Lychees	Pomegranates	Tejocotes

Excluded Avocados, bananas, citrus or citrus zest, dates, figs, pineapple, papayas, passion fruit, raspberries, raisins, red plums

Notes
- Dried fruits (except raisins) are OK as long as they do not contain sulfites.
- Fresh fruits on the list may be dried in a home dehydrator.

Sweetener

Approved Stevia (without any additives, even raw sugar)

Excluded Sugar, honey, maple or other syrups, artificial sweeteners, sugar alcohols like xylitol or maltitol

Protein (should be fresh and freshly cooked)

Approved			
Beans (except exclusions)	Fish (fresh or frozen without coatings or seasonings)	Salmon (if canned, Wild Alaskan with no salt or other additives)	Shellfish (no salt, sodium, or other additives)
Beef (grass-fed/pastured)	Pork (pastured)		Tuna (if canned, no salt or other additives)
Eggs (local, free-range)	Poultry (free-range)	Seeds (sunflower, flax, chia, sesame, hemp)	

Excluded Dried or smoked fish, smoked or preserved meats (like sausage), favas, limas, navy beans, soybeans, lentils

Notes
- Uncured reduced-sodium pastured bacon can be tested after four months.

Dairy

Approved			
American cheese	Cottage cheese	Cream cheese	Milk
Chèvre (fresh goat cheese)	Cream	Mascarpone	Ricotta

Excluded Hard, aged cheeses, processed cheese

Notes
- If you can find American cheese that is organic and soy-free, most lists include it as OK. It's not recommended for Meniere's because of its high sodium content. The plastic-wrapped "singles" are not OK.

Fats and oils (organic extra virgin if possible)

Approved	Butter (organic, grass-fed, and unsalted)	Lard or rendered bacon fat (from pastured pigs)	Sesame oil (regular and toasted in small amounts)	Tallow (beef fat from grass-fed cows)
	Coconut oil	Olive oil	Sunflower seed oil (in small amounts)	
Excluded	Trans fats; corn, cottonseed, canola, rapeseed, soybean, peanut, nut oils			

Herbs, spices, and condiments

Approved	All herbs (except exclusions)	All spices (except exclusions)	Clear, white vinegar (limited to ½ teaspoon per recipe)
Excluded	Spice blends containing MSG, salt, seaweed or seaweed extracts (including kombu, nori, hijiki, carrageenan, and agar agar), "flavorings," onion powder, yeast, nutritional yeast, store-bought condiments, salad dressings, and vinegar other than organic white vinegar		

Notes
- Some people may be sensitive to paprika, smoked paprika, chili powder, and curry powders containing chili powder.
- Even white vinegar can be a trigger, so limit consumption.
- After four months on the Plan, you can test apple cider vinegar, rice wine vinegar, white balsamic, and white wine vinegar.
- Use the smallest amount possible in recipes, unless you are positive that vinegar isn't a trigger.

Drinks

Approved	Coconut milk	Hemp milk	Infused water	Vodka (small amounts)
	Coconut water	Herbal teas (except exclusions)	Milk	White wine (small amounts)
	Filtered or spring water		Sparkling water (without citrus flavoring)	
Excluded	Nut milks; boxed milks that include carrageenan or gums; soy milk; red wine; hard liquors; beer; soda (regular or diet); caffeinated tea; herbal tea containing citrus, raspberry, or hibiscus; caffeinated coffee			

Notes
- Do not use wine in cooking for the first four months, then test it for yourself.
- Besides being a powerful migraine trigger, coffee also raises cortisol levels for up to six hours. Elevated cortisol levels can lead to an overactive immune system, sleep disruptions and impairment, and depression.
- Decaf coffee is OK but might still be a trigger.

At a Glance: The No List

Common triggers

Aged foods and cheeses	Condiments	Nutritional yeast	Soy products
Avocados	Cured meats	Nuts	Soy sauce
Bananas	Dried fish	Salad dressings	Vinegars
Citrus and most tropical fruits	Fermented foods (sauerkraut, miso, kombucha, kefir)	Seaweed	

Additives that are triggers

Autolyzed yeast	Glutamic acid	Natural flavors/flavorings	Textured vegetable protein
Calcium caseinate	Hydrolyzed protein	Protein-fortified items	Ultra-pasteurized items
Carrageenan	Kombu (seaweed extract)	Sodium caseinate	Whey protein and any protein powder
Enzyme-modified items	Malt extract	Soy protein concentrate/isolate	Yeast extract
Fermented or cultured items	Malted barley	Store-bought broth, stock, bouillon	
Gelatin (grass-fed gelatin is OK)	Maltodextrin		
	MSG		

Notes   Visit truthinlabeling.org to find a longer list of potential names for soy additives.

Hidden sugars

Agave nectar or syrup	Crystalline fructose	Inulin	Sorbitol
Barley malt or syrup	Date sugar	Jaggery	Sorghum molasses or syrup
Beet sugar	Dextrin	Lactitol, lactose	Sucrose
Brown rice, rice bran syrup	Dextrose	Malt or malted syrup	Sugar or syrup (brown, demerara, invert, muscovado, palm, rapidura, raw cane, sucanat, turbinado)
Cane crystals, juice, or syrup (dehydrated/evaporated)	Ethyl maltitol	Maltodextrin	
	Fructose	Maltose	
	Fruit juice concentrate	Mannitol	
Coconut (sugar)	Galactose	Maple syrup, sugar	Treacle
Corn (sugar, syrup, solids)	Glucose (syrup, solids)	Molasses	Yacon
	Golden syrup	Monk fruit (luo han guo)	
Corn syrup (solids), high-fructose corn syrup	Honey	Mono- or Oligosaccharide	
	Hydrogenated or hydrolyzed starch	Panela, panocha	
		Saccharose	

Notes   Watch out for anything with the words sugar, granulated, syrup, saccharide, and crystal, and any ingredients with an –ose at the end of them.

What You Need to Know

Recipe instructions assume that produce has been washed and that alliums such as onions, garlic cloves, and shallots have been peeled. Recipes calling for root vegetables like carrots and potatoes should be scrubbed but not peeled, unless otherwise specified. All recipes using green onions (otherwise known as scallions) use the white and green portions together unless otherwise indicated. All recipes use large, free-range eggs and large garlic cloves. Recipes calling for coconut milk use full-fat canned coconut milk unless otherwise specified. I use the more common term *broth*, rather than *stock*, to refer to vegetable or chicken broth. Butter is unsalted, grass-fed, and organic, if possible. Whenever possible, meat is grass-fed, chicken is free-range, vegetables and fruit are organic, canned goods such as broth, tomatoes, and beans are no-salt-added or low-sodium, and dried fruit is unsweetened and unsulphured. Where I call for white vinegar, I recommend using organic distilled white vinegar (free of GMO corn). Check the Shopping Guide on the next page for more information about specific ingredients.

If you know you are sensitive to an ingredient, like stevia or chipotle pepper, you will need to make a substitution to any recipe containing that ingredient.

NUTRITIONAL INFORMATION: I chose not to include calorie counts for the recipes, because focusing on calories is not the most helpful way to look at food. (Please see pages 149 and 150 of *The Migraine Relief Plan* for a thorough explanation.) Recipe analysis is provided for people who need to track macronutrients like carbohydrates or fat, or specifics like sodium, potassium, or saturated fat.

BUDGET-FRIENDLY INDICATORS: Recipes are listed as Very or Moderate, meaning that ingredients are readily available and less expensive (Very) or a bit more expensive or available online, where there may be a shipping cost (Moderate).

TIME INDICATORS: Prep Time includes time spent organizing ingredients, preparing raw ingredients (peeling, chopping, slicing), and/or stirring before cooking. Cook Time includes all active cooking time on the stove or in the oven. Passive Time includes any additional time needed to soak, marinate, or cool.

DIETARY ICONS: For readers who follow a special diet or have food sensitivities, I've created icons for each recipe. A recipe includes that icon if it can be made to fit that diet: Vegan/Vegetarian, Dairy-Free, Egg-Free, and Grain-Free. All recipes are gluten-free, free of processed sugar, free of added salt, and anti-inflammatory.

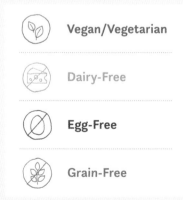

Vegan/Vegetarian

Dairy-Free

Egg-Free

Grain-Free

Shopping Guide

Choose organic versions of the following whenever possible:

Arrowroot powder: A finely ground white powder made from the tuber of the arrowroot plant. Used as a starch or thickener in gluten-free and paleo recipes. Can substitute in recipes calling for cornstarch if you are avoiding corn. Use double the amount to get the same results you would with cornstarch. (If thickening a sauce or a filling that will be baked, like a pie, I prefer using tapioca flour or starch as it yields a firmer result.)

Baking soda substitute, sodium-free: A leavening agent used in baking. Traditional baking soda is made from bicarbonate of soda and is therefore a salt; baking soda substitute, such as Ener-G, is a mixture of calcium carbonate and magnesium carbonate. Use double the amount of regular baking powder or baking soda as called for.

Carob powder: The ground pods of an evergreen tree. Used as a chocolate substitute. (Don't expect it to taste exactly like chocolate, but rather chocolate-like.) Naturally sweet, low in fat, high in calcium, and caffeine-free.

Chipotle chili powder: Ground, smoked, dried jalapeños. Might be a migraine trigger, so use sparingly until you rule it out. Doesn't take much to add spicy, smoky flavor to foods like chili. Start with ⅛ teaspoon.

Coconut milk: Made from coconut and water. Some brands include gums and other thickeners that might be triggers. Check the ingredients list. Guar gum should be okay. My recipes call for full-fat canned coconut milk unless specifically noted.

Coconut oil: A fat derived from coconut. Extra-virgin is best; you can use refined organic coconut oil for high-heat frying or to avoid adding coconut flavor.

Coconut sugar: Sap from the coconut palm tree is boiled until it forms crystals. Coconut sugar retains some nutrients from the sap, including trace amounts of iron, zinc, calcium, and potassium, along with some short-chain fatty acids like polyphenols and antioxidants. Unlike white sugar, it contains a fiber called inulin, which may slow glucose absorption and explains why coconut sugar has a lower glycemic index than regular white sugar.

Curry powder: Refers to a variety of similar, yellow-hued spice blends sold in US grocery stores, usually labeled mild, medium, or hot, and generally containing some combination of cumin, turmeric, pepper, ginger, and other spices. No-salt-added versions are sold by Penzeys and Spicely Organics. Not an Indian ingredient, curry powder was invented by the British. You will find versions of spice blends and mixes used in Thai, Burmese, Malaysian, Indonesian, or Singaporean curries in specialty and gourmet spice stores. Check the ingredients list. If they do not contain salt or MSG, they can be used on the Plan if the heat level is comfortable for your palate.

Dried mustard: Made of ground mustard seeds, this stands in for jarred mustard, which contains sodium, vinegar, and other possible triggers.

Extra-virgin olive oil: To be designated extra-virgin, the oil must be pressed without the use of heat or chemicals and must be from the first pressing of the olives. Usually dark green or yellow-green in color, it is unrefined. Buy in small quantities and store in the refrigerator or away from heat and light. Use it raw to maintain the highest health benefits from the polyphenol compounds. Light olive oil is refined and is light yellow in color. I use it for making mayonnaise; it's also good for cooking if you don't care for the taste of coconut oil or animal fat, or if you want to save money.

Filtered water: I only use filtered water when I cook. It offers three benefits: 1) It removes many harmful minerals and chemicals that might be in your tap water. 2) It tastes better than tap water. 3) It removes sodium from the water. Spring water also works.

Ghee: Clarified butter used in Indian cooking, with milk proteins removed. Good for high heat cooking and for people with milk-protein allergies or sensitivities. Choose grass-fed organic ghee if available.

Gluten-free flour blend: Use a blend with at least four flours, including tapioca starch, and a binder like xanthan gum. Some people are sensitive to xanthan gum.

Psyllium husk powder: A high-fiber seed that absorbs water at a magical rate. Helps bind gluten-free dough and prevents it from crumbling. I use it, with great results, substituted one for one in recipes that call for xanthan gum. Look for it in the health food stores; it is also widely available at online markets.

Quinoa: A high-protein, gluten-free grain alternative, available in black, tan, red, or mixed varieties. When cooked, grains have a tiny curly tail. Another good substitute for couscous or bulgur wheat. Rinse and drain before cooking.

Sea salt: Commercial white table salt contains potassium iodide, dextrose, and sodium bicarbonate; bleach is used during the refining process, and it may also contain sugar. It may be implicated in auto-immune conditions. Natural sea salt contains as many as eighty elements in trace amounts. Look for natural sea salt in any color (pink, grey, blue) and use sparingly at the table.

Smoked paprika: Also called pimenton, it's a type of paprika—a spice made from ground red peppers—that is smoked and dried. It provides delicious smoky flavor. It is available in sweet and hot varieties. Peppers and smoked foods are a trigger for some. I use it in small amounts.

Stevia: A natural sweetener from the leaves of the stevia plant, this is far sweeter than sugar. For the best taste, choose an organic brand without added fillers like erythritol or xylitol. Most stevia packets are the equivalent of 2 teaspoons sugar, but this varies by brand and whether they have fillers. With liquid stevia, 5 drops is usually the equivalent of 1 teaspoon sugar. If you cannot use stevia, substitute coconut sugar in the amount called for in the recipe. You might find that growing the plant itself will improve your experience of stevia. Use fresh leaves to sweeten iced tea, and dried powdered leaves in recipes in very small amounts.

Tahini: Sesame seeds crushed into a creamy paste. Used in hummus, it is also used in marinades and salad dressings to amp up the sesame flavor. Usually contains no additional ingredients. Store in the refrigerator.

Tapioca starch: Also labeled tapioca flour. Get the finest grind you can; you want it as powdery as flour, not grainy.

Toasted sesame oil: Also labeled dark toasted sesame oil. Adds savory, rich flavor to marinades and stir fry dishes, especially in the absence of soy.

"Our pain, our illnesses, our losses, our injuries, they are part of who we are. I really believe that we only grow when we pay attention to these very hard experiences. The first step in post-traumatic growth is to acknowledge the suffering and be honest with ourselves and others."

DR. MICHAELA HAAS, AUTHOR OF *BOUNCING FORWARD: THE ART AND SCIENCE OF CULTIVATING RESILIENCE*

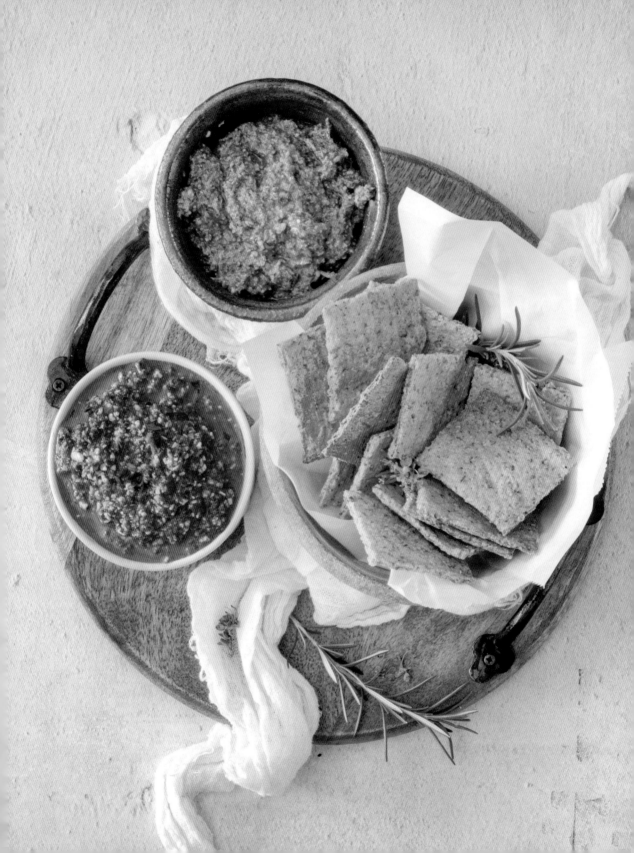

Snacks

When I surveyed readers to find out what recipes they needed more of, snacks topped the list. They wanted more dips, more on-the-go options, and a lower-carb smoothie so they could more easily stay on the Plan. Packaged snack foods tend to be high in sodium, which can be an issue for those of us with vertigo. They also tend to contain sugar and seed oils high in omega-6 fatty acids such as soybean, corn, and cottonseed, which may contribute to inflammation.

Trail Mix

If you love to hike and camp, or want an on-the-go snack to eat in the car or at your desk, this recipe is for you. I combine sweet, natural coconut with toasted seeds and dried Bing cherries for the perfect combination of hearty and sweet.

Makes 16 servings

Prep time: 5 minutes
Cooking time: N/A
Passive time: N/A

Budget friendly: Moderate

1 cup (50g) unsweetened flaked coconut

1 cup (120g) toasted pumpkin seeds, no salt added

1 cup (130g) toasted sunflower seeds, no salt added

1 cup (165g) unsweetened and unsulphured dried Bing cherries

1 Mix all the ingredients together in a large bowl.

2 Store in an airtight container for up to 3 weeks.

COOK'S NOTE: *As you test your tolerance for nuts, raisins, and chocolate, you can substitute these items to make your own unique blend. I recommend Lily's stevia-sweetened chocolate chips. If you aren't too sensitive to sodium, use salted, toasted sunflower seeds. Dried Bing cherries may be found at Trader Joe's; they are also available online. The effort is worth it, as they add a necessary sweetness.*

PER ¼-CUP SERVING: 4g protein, 10g carbohydrates, 9g fat, 3g saturated fat, 95mg sodium, 103mg potassium, 2g fiber

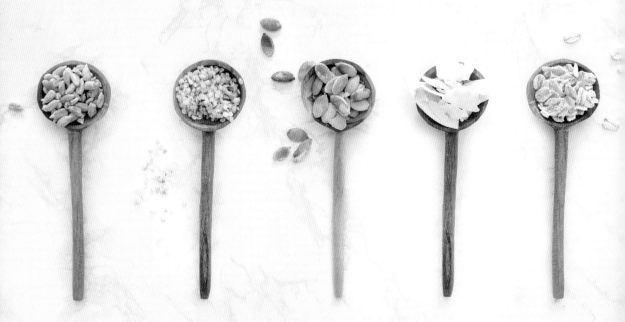

Chewy Cherry Oat Bars

One of the biggest challenges in following a special diet is that very few packaged snacks fit your plan. I created these to meet your needs for on-the-go healthy snacks, since you can toss them in a purse or backpack. To make them low in added sugar, the sweetness comes from the dried cherries, which also provide an anti-oxidant boost. These are lower in carbohydrates than many sugary store-bought bars, and much higher in protein due to the seeds and eggs.

Makes 10 bars

Prep time: 10 minutes
Cooking time: 12 minutes
Passive time: 30 minutes

Budget friendly: Moderate

1 cup (165g) unsweetened and unsulphured dried Bing cherries, cut into smaller pieces

¾ cup (100g) sunflower seeds

½ cup (50g) rolled oats

½ cup (80g) shelled hemp seeds

¼ cup (32g) sesame seeds

3 eggs

1 tablespoon extra-virgin olive or melted coconut oil

20 drops vanilla stevia extract (optional)

1 Preheat oven to 350°F (180°C). Prepare a baking sheet by lining it with parchment paper, a silicone mat, or oiling lightly.

2 Place all the ingredients in a large bowl and mix well.

3 Using a wide spatula, smooth mixture into an even layer on the prepared baking sheet, making an 8½-inch × 10-inch (22cm × 25cm) rectangle.

4 Bake 12 minutes, or until lightly browned on the edges and firm to the touch in the center.

5 Let cool for 30 minutes on a wire rack, then cut into 10 (2-inch × 4¼-inch [5cm × 11cm]) bars.

6 Store in the refrigerator or freezer in zip-top bags.

COOK'S NOTE: *Unsulphured apricots or soft, dried mango can be substituted for the cherries. Shelled hemp seeds, also called hemp hearts, are available in many grocery stores, as well as online markets. Do not use shell-on hemp seeds. Be sure to store seeds in the refrigerator or freezer since they don't contain preservatives and will spoil faster when exposed to heat and light.*

PER SERVING: 8g protein, 16g carbohydrates, 13g fat, 3g saturated fat, 21mg sodium, 120mg potassium, 3g fiber

Blueberry Muffins

This recipe was inspired by a favorite podcast, *The Satellite Sisters*. The hosts are real-life sisters whose mother, Edna Dolan, made blueberry muffins every Fourth of July from a recipe she adapted from the *New York Times*. Bursting with fresh or frozen blueberries, they make a terrific snack plain or slathered with butter, served with your favorite cup of tea.

Makes 12 generously sized muffins

Prep time: 15 minutes
Cooking time: 25–28 minutes
Passive time: 15 minutes for cooling

Budget friendly: Very

1¾ cups (260g) gluten-free flour such as Bob's Red Mill 1-to-1 Baking Flour or my Gluten-Free Flour Blend (p. 203), sifted

1 tablespoon regular or sodium-free baking powder

¼ cup plus 2 tablespoons (60g) coconut sugar, plus more for sprinkling

Stevia to equal 3 teaspoons sugar

3 eggs

½ cup (118mL) whole, hemp, or coconut milk

¼ cup (59mL) olive oil or 4 tablespoons melted butter

2½ cups (375g) blueberries, fresh or frozen

1 Preheat oven to 425°F (220°C). Line muffin tins with 12 paper liners or place silicone muffin liners on a baking sheet.

2 In a medium bowl, whisk the flour, baking powder, sugar, and Stevia together until well combined.

3 In a large bowl, beat the eggs with a hand or stand mixer fitted with the paddle attachment for three minutes until thick and creamy. Stir in the milk and olive oil, then stir in the flour mixture until just combined. Do not overmix.

4 Carefully fold in the berries.

5 Distribute the batter evenly in the lined muffin tins.

6 Sprinkle lightly with additional coconut sugar.

7 Place the muffin tins on the middle rack of the oven.

8 Bake for 25 to 28 minutes, or until the muffins are golden brown and tops are cracked.

9 Remove muffins from the tins and cool on wire racks.

COOK'S NOTE: *Sift or fluff the flour before measuring. I get the best baking results from Bob's Red Mill Gluten-Free 1-to-1 Baking Flour. If you cannot find it, or if you want to try homemade, use my Gluten-Free Flour Blend (p. 203). If the blend you buy does not include xanthan gum or psyllium husk powder, whisk 2 teaspoons xanthan gum or psyllium husk powder into the dry ingredients in Step 2. Organic cane sugar can be substituted for the coconut sugar. Very large blueberries will produce delicious but unevenly shaped muffins.*

 If buttermilk is not a trigger for you, use it in place of the milk for incredible results.

PER SERVING (with olive oil, hemp milk, and sodium-free baking powder):
3g protein, 28g carbohydrates, 6g fat, 1g saturated fat, 29mg sodium, 41mg potassium, 1g fiber

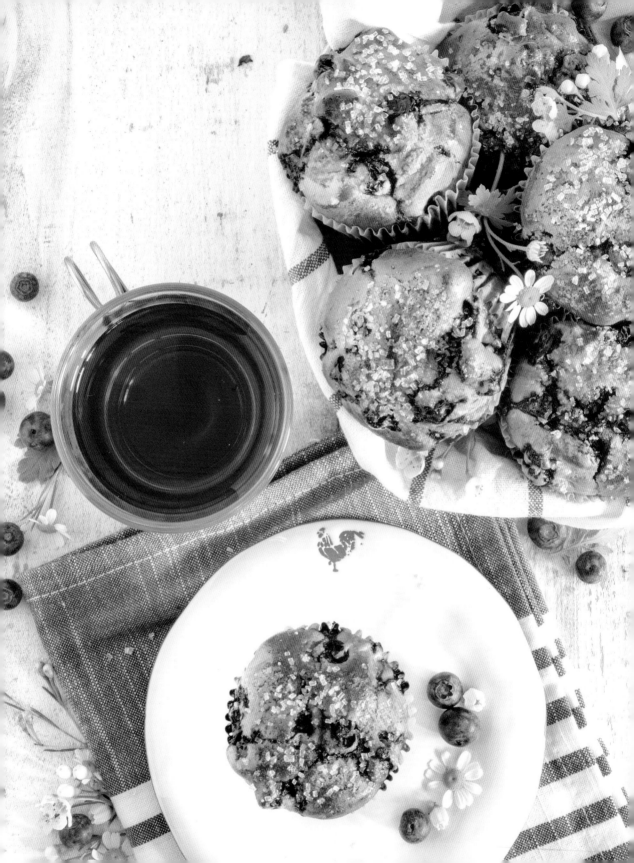

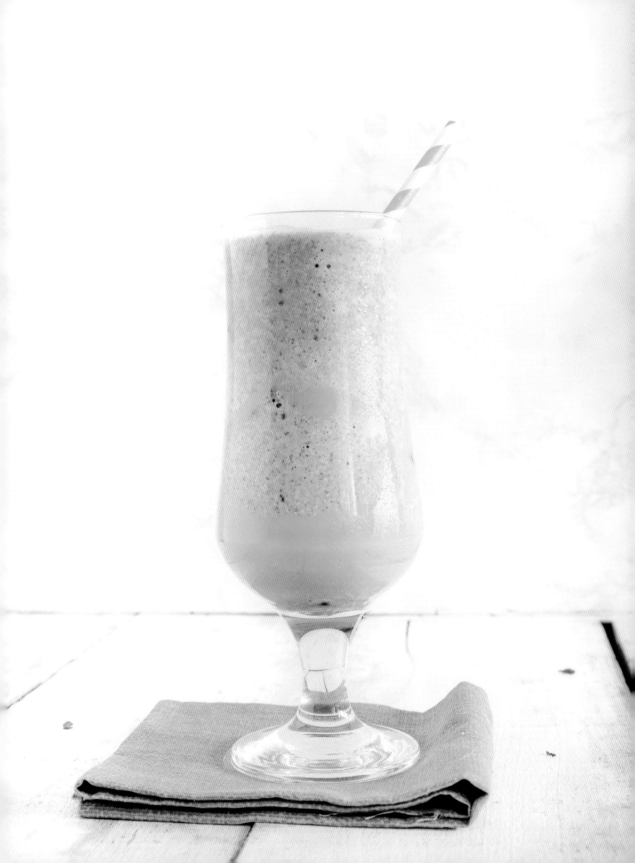

Shamrock Smoothie

I've never had a McDonald's Shamrock Shake, which is a milkshake loaded with sugars like high-fructose corn syrup. Instead, I've created this Shamrock Smoothie, packed with protein from three kinds of seeds, with no added sugar. The bright green color comes from fresh spinach, not food coloring, and I use organic peppermint extract and a small amount of stevia to give it a fresh, minty flavor.

Makes 1 smoothie

Prep time: 3 minutes
Cooking time: N/A
Passive time: N/A

Budget friendly: Moderate

¾ cup (180mL) whole, hemp, or coconut milk

1 tablespoon hemp seeds

1 tablespoon chia seeds

1 tablespoon sunflower seed butter

Stevia to equal 2 teaspoons sugar

⅛ teaspoon alcohol-free peppermint extract

4–5 ice cubes

2 large handfuls baby spinach

1 With the blender running, add ingredients in the order listed.

2 Blend until smooth and creamy. Smoothie will thicken as it sits.

COOK'S NOTE: *Avoid non-dairy milk containing guar gum, xanthan gum, and carrageenan. Consider making your own hemp milk (p. 255,* The Migraine Relief Plan).

PER SERVING: 12g protein, 11g carbohydrates, 22g fat, 2g saturated fat, 115mg sodium, 402mg potassium, 8g fiber

Creamy Not-ella Carob Butter

This easy, rich-tasting treat was my favorite recipe in *The Migraine Relief Plan*. I'm sharing it here because it's an ingredient in the Choco-Berry Sorbet (p. 178). Whip up a jar to smear on gluten-free toast, rice cakes, or sliced apples for a sweet snack. The commercial varieties of hazelnut-chocolate spreads include allergens like hazelnuts and milk, are high in sugar, and contain trans fats. Since nuts and chocolate are not on the Plan, I've substituted toasted sunflower seeds and hemp seeds for the hazelnuts, carob powder for the cocoa, and use coconut oil and stevia to create the rich flavor.

Makes 16 servings

Prep time: 10–15 minutes
Cooking time: 20–30 minutes
Passive time: 15 minutes

Budget friendly: Moderate

1 cup (230g) sunflower seeds

1 cup (160g) hemp seeds

Stevia to equal 8 teaspoons sugar

½ cup (50g) carob powder

4 tablespoons (60mL) coconut oil, melted

1 Preheat the oven to 300°F (150°C). Put the sunflower seeds on a baking sheet lined with fresh parchment paper.

2 Toast the sunflower seeds for 10 minutes, then stir and return to the oven. Turn off the oven and toast the seeds another 5 to 10 minutes. Check every few minutes, until the seeds are just barely golden brown but not burnt. Taste a few if you aren't sure.

3 Let the toasted sunflower seeds cool for 15 minutes.

4 Put the toasted seeds in a food processor fitted with the S-blade or a high-speed blender and blend into a fine powder, about a minute.

5 Add the hemp seeds and stevia and blend for about 4 more minutes. Pause every minute to scrape down the sides. Eventually a ball will form and become the consistency of nut butter.

6 Blend the carob powder with the oil in a separate bowl, then add to the sunflower seed butter and blend until smooth. (If you add the carob powder and oil directly to the food processor, you will have a powdery carob explosion that is not fun to clean up.)

7 Place the carob butter in a glass jar and store in the refrigerator. It will be spreadable when refrigerated, and just a little thicker than chocolate-hazelnut spread at room temperature.

COOK'S NOTE: *If you cannot find shelled hemp seeds, also called hemp hearts, sunflower seeds are a good substitute. Do not use shell-on hemp seeds in this recipe.*

PER 1-OUNCE SERVING: 5g protein, 9g carbohydrates, 11g fat, 3g saturated fat, 6mg sodium, 61mg potassium, 2g fiber

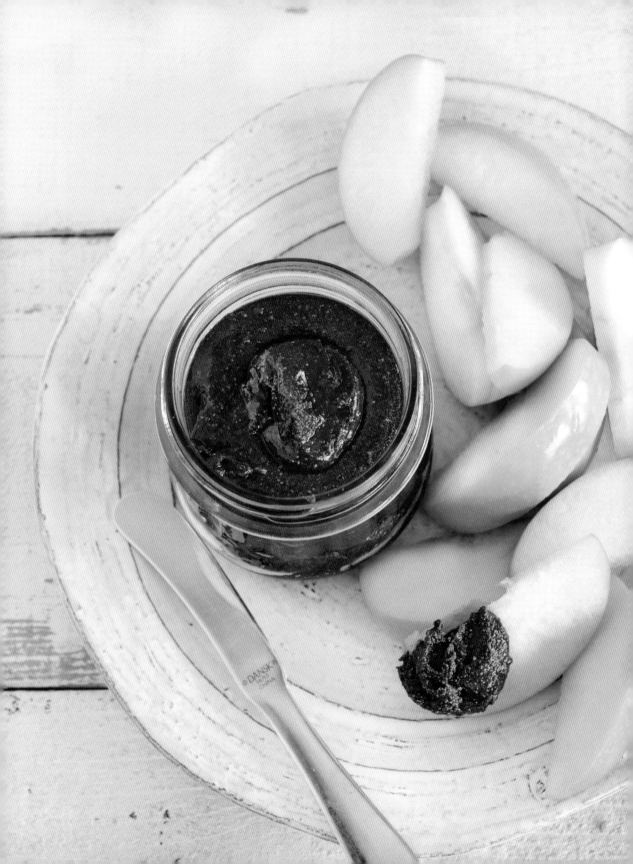

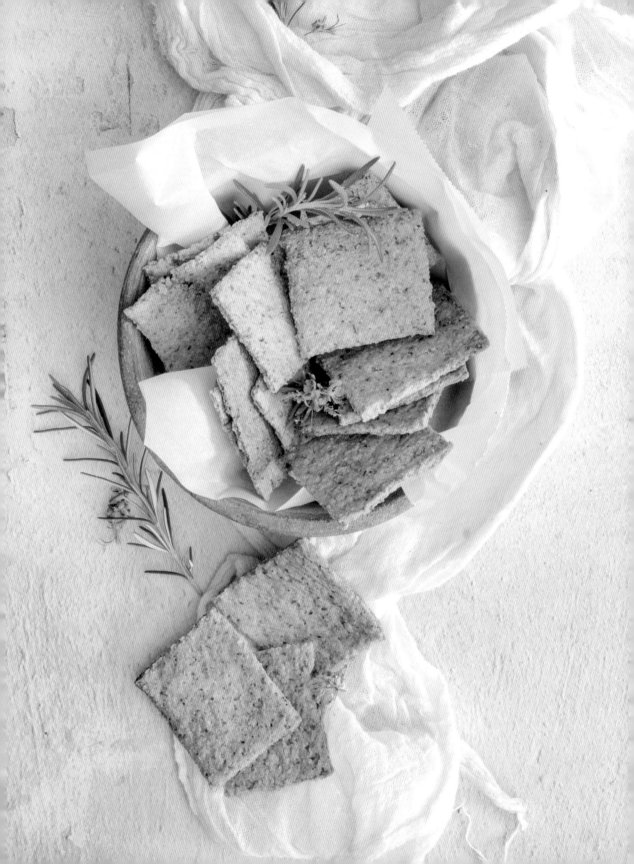

Herbed Olive Oil Crackers

Crackers that follow the Plan are difficult to find. I had never considered making my own, but it's surprisingly easy. Roll these out as thinly as possible to create a crispy cracker. Skip the salt if you're following a super-low-sodium diet.

Makes 54 small crackers

Prep time: 20 minutes
Cooking time: 20–23 minutes
Passive time: 30 minutes

Budget friendly: Very

2 tablespoons ground flax seeds

½ cup (125mL) filtered water

1 cup (120g) oat flour

½ cup (65g) toasted sunflower seeds, pulsed to a fine meal in a food processor

2 tablespoons extra-virgin olive oil

2 tablespoons hemp, light coconut, or whole milk

1 tablespoon no-salt-added Italian herb or another spice blend

1 teaspoon sodium-free baking soda substitute (see Shopping Guide on p. 17)

⅛ teaspoon fine sea salt (optional)

SERVING SUGGESTIONS: Serve with Curried Cilantro Pesto (p. 34), Roasted Red Pepper Romesco-Style Dip (p. 32), Herbed Cheese Spread (p. 189, *The Migraine Relief Plan*), Roasted Chile Pepper Hummus (p. 190, *The Migraine Relief Plan*).

1 Preheat the oven to 425°F (220°C).

2 Place the flax seeds in a mixing bowl with the water to thicken. Leave for at least 5 minutes.

3 Cut a piece of parchment paper the size of a large baking sheet, 12-inch × 14-inch (30cm × 35cm). Set aside.

4 Add the rest of the ingredients, except the fine sea salt, to the mixing bowl. Blend by hand or with a stand mixer fitted with the paddle attachment until the dough is sticky and smooth.

5 Set the dough on the prepared parchment paper and top with a piece of plastic wrap. Press the dough into a rough circle by hand, then use a rolling pin to roll it thinly to the edges of the paper. Remove plastic wrap.

6 Move the dough (still on the paper) to the baking sheet. Sprinkle with salt if using.

7 With a pizza cutter or sharp knife, completely score the dough, through to the paper, into small rectangles. To get 54 crackers, score the long side into 8 equal parts and the shorter side into 7.

8 Bake 20 to 23 minutes, or until the crackers are golden brown and very crispy. Rotate pan halfway through.

9 Transfer to a wire rack. When completely cool, carefully separate the crackers and store in an airtight container.

COOK'S NOTE: *Substitute gluten-free sorghum or brown rice flour for the oat flour. If you are not following a low-sodium diet, use regular baking soda. Herbes de Provence, chili powder, or curry powder may be substituted for the Italian herb blend. If you cannot find toasted, no-salt-added sunflower seeds, follow the method on p. 28.*

PER 6 CRACKERS: 5g protein, 14g carbohydrates, 9g fat, 1g saturated fat, 32mg sodium, 100mg potassium, 3g fiber

Roasted Red Pepper Romesco-Style Dip

Romesco sauce is a roasted pepper sauce thickened with bread. It is a Spanish staple that originated in Catalonia. True romesco is made with almonds, tomatoes, and paprika. I made this Plan-friendly version because the sauce is so versatile—it can be used as a dip for vegetables, a spread for sandwiches, and a sauce for red meat, chicken, and seafood.

Makes 12 servings

Prep time: 5 minutes
Cooking time: 15 minutes
Passive time: 15 minutes

Budget friendly: Very

1½ medium red bell peppers, about 12 ounces (340g)

1 unpeeled garlic clove (optional)

3 ounces (45g) toasted sunflower seeds

3 tablespoons fresh Italian parsley, minced

2 tablespoons extra-virgin olive oil

½ teaspoon white vinegar

¼ teaspoon freshly ground black pepper

¼ teaspoon garlic powder (if not using fresh garlic)

1 Cut the peppers in half and remove and discard the core, seeds, and ribs. Cut slits to flatten, and press the peppers face down onto a baking sheet. Add the unpeeled garlic clove to the pan, if using.

2 Broil for 10 minutes, or until the peppers are evenly blackened and the skin is blistered.

3 With tongs, place the peppers and garlic in a paper bag and roll the top closed. Let sit for at least 15 minutes to cool.

4 Peel the blackened skin from the peppers. Discard the skin.

5 Place all the ingredients in a food processor or blender. If you broiled a garlic clove, squeeze the center into the machine, and discard the papery skin.

6 Pulse until romesco reaches desired consistency—smooth for a sauce and chunky for a dip. Store in the refrigerator and use within 3 days.

COOK'S NOTE: *Substitute jarred roasted red peppers for quicker preparation; be sure to drain the peppers first. If you cannot find toasted, no-salt-added sunflower seeds, follow the method on p. 28.*

SERVING SUGGESTIONS: Romesco is lovely as a condiment on grilled fish or poultry, or as a dip with Herbed Olive Oil Crackers (p. 31) or Seedy Carrot Crackers (p. 192, *The Migraine Relief Plan*).

PER 1-OUNCE SERVING: 2g protein, 3g carbohydrates, 6g fat, 1g saturated fat, 3mg sodium, 72mg potassium, 1g fiber

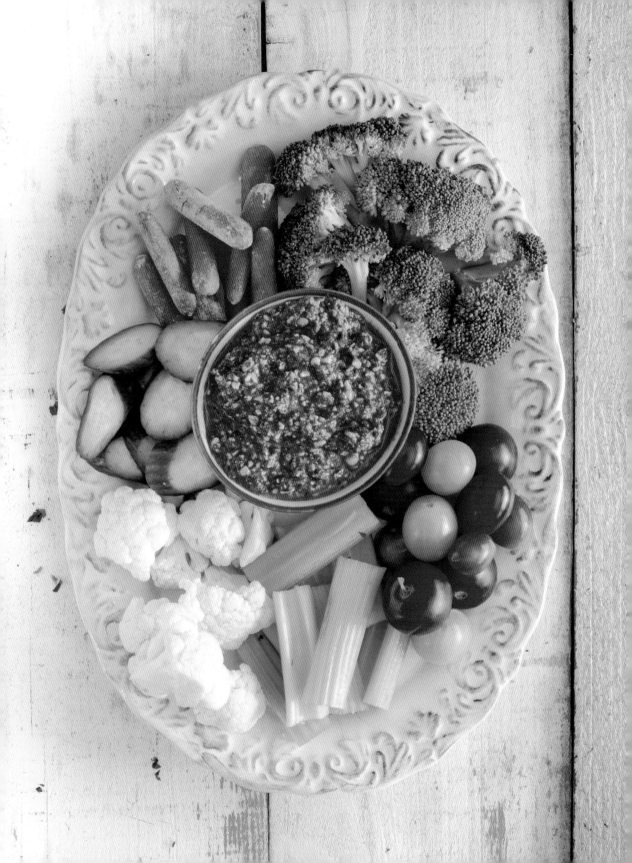

Curried Cilantro Pesto

Rich and garlicky, this versatile spread is a perfect party dip. If you use it as a sauce, know it's free of the artificial ingredients and high sodium levels found in many store-bought dips. Plan-friendly hemp seeds stand in for the pine nuts found in traditional pesto.

Makes about 6 servings

Prep time:	5 minutes
Cooking time:	N/A
Passive time:	N/A

Budget friendly: Very

2 cups packed (3.5 ounces [100g]) cilantro, washed, dried well in a kitchen towel

1 small clove garlic

4 tablespoons (60mL) extra-virgin olive oil

4 tablespoons (40g) raw hemp seeds

1 teaspoon medium no-salt-added curry powder (See Cook's Note)

1 Use kitchen scissors to trim and discard the ends of the cilantro stems. Cut the cilantro bunch iinto pieces and add to the bowl of a food processor.

2 Add the garlic, olive oil, hemp seeds, and curry powder.

3 Process, stopping to scrape down the sides once or twice. If necessary, add more olive oil to achieve your desired consistency. When I toss it with pasta, I make it loose and a little runny by adding more olive oil. When I serve it as a dip or spread, I make it thicker.

4 Store in the refrigerator and use within 3 days or freeze in small containers.

COOK'S NOTE: *If you do not like cilantro, substitute Italian flat-leaf parsley. When I call for curry powder, I am referring to the spice blend sold in US supermarkets, generally labeled mild, medium, or hot, and sometimes labeled "Madras Curry Powder." Choose a no-salt-added blend. Curry powder means different things to the cuisines and cultures that use the term. It's not an Indian term, as Indian dishes call for turmeric and other spices blended specifically for a dish.*

SERVING SUGGESTIONS: Serve with Herbed Olive Oil Crackers (p. 31), Seedy Carrot Crackers (p. 192, *The Migraine Relief Plan*), hearty rice cakes, or toss with gluten-free pasta. Serve as a dip with raw vegetables, spread on a sandwich, or use as a sauce for meat, poultry, or fish.

PER 2-TABLESPOON SERVING:
3g protein, 1g carbohydrates, 12g fat, 2g saturated fat, 8mg sodium, 153mg potassium, 1g fiber

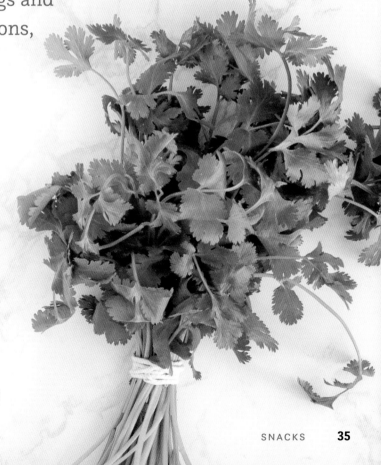

"When life tries to knock you down, you learn to either not fall or not fall as far. You don't have to see it as, 'Okay, now I have to recover again. I have to learn how to be this person who's constantly recovering.' Shame and guilt, there's no place for that. We don't need them. We need to learn to just say no to those emotions. And I think that plays a big role in resilience, because if we're able to say no to these negative feelings and these negative emotions, we don't get knocked down as far."

**LINDSAY WEITZEL, PH.D.,
MIGRAINE STRATEGIST**

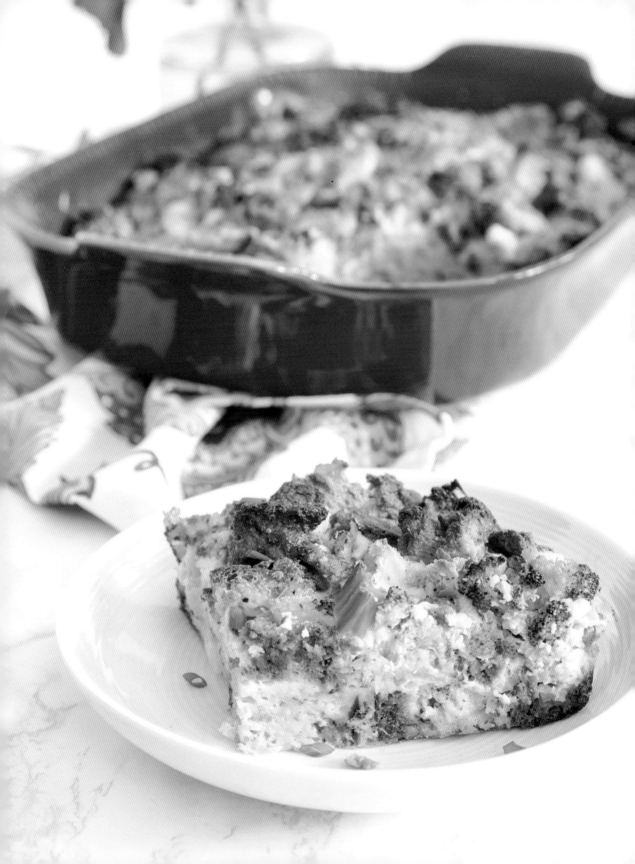

Breakfast

It is important to eat in the morning, as low blood sugar is known to be a migraine trigger. If you're not used to eating first thing, small portions are fine. I've offered weekend brunch ideas, recipes to incorporate vegetables into your first meal of the day, and a portable egg dish you can make in the microwave.

Breakfast Hash

My husband and I eat some version of this hash nearly every day. I love starting the day with a serving of vegetables. I dice extra veggies when I cook on the weekend and freeze them in zip-top bags. This allows me to quickly make a new batch with ingredients straight from the freezer.

Makes 6 servings

Prep time: 15 minutes
Cooking time: 20 minutes
Passive time: N/A

Budget friendly: Very

2 tablespoons extra-virgin olive oil

1 large carrot, diced

1 medium sweet potato, peeled and diced

¼ head (175g) cabbage, red or green, thinly sliced

1 stalk broccoli, stem peeled and diced, florets separated

1 Heat the oil in a large skillet or nonstick sauté pan over medium heat.

2 When the oil is shimmering, tilt the pan until it is evenly coated, and add all the vegetables except for the broccoli florets. Stir.

3 Cook, stirring every couple of minutes, for 12 to 15 minutes, until the carrot and sweet potato are tender and can be pierced with a fork.

4 Add the broccoli florets and cook until just bright green.

COOK'S NOTE: *Many other sliced or diced vegetables will work, including kale, cauliflower, green onions, bell pepper, brussels sprouts, jicama, rutabaga, celery, and beets. You must use a large skillet or sauté pan for this recipe, otherwise the vegetables will steam and not caramelize properly.*

SERVING SUGGESTIONS: Top hash with a single, over-easy or poached egg and serve with Turkey Sausage Patties (p. 51), Make Your Own Bacon (p. 197, *The Migraine Relief Plan*), or Pork Sausage Patties (p. 208, *The Migraine Relief Plan*).

PER SERVING: 1g protein, 9g carbohydrates, 5g fat, 1g saturated fat, 33mg sodium, 244mg potassium, 2g fiber

Quickie Microwave Egg Scramble

This scramble makes a healthy breakfast that can be prepared with the appliances available in most workplace kitchens. Prep the ingredients over the weekend and pack them in advance. (Put the first 4 ingredients in a container with a lid and pack the egg separately so it doesn't break.) This is a great way to use up leftover cooked meat and vegetables.

Makes 1 serving

Prep time: 5 minutes
Cooking time: 2–3 minutes
Passive time: N/A

Budget friendly: Very

¼ cup (42g) cooked potato, finely diced

¼ cup (40g) sautéed peppers, finely diced

¼ cup (63g) ricotta cheese

3–4 tablespoons (18–25g) cooked Turkey Sausage Patties (p. 51), finely crumbled

1 egg

1 Place all the ingredients in a microwave-safe glass container or coffee mug. Stir well, breaking the yolk.

2 Microwave on full power for 40 seconds. Stir.

3 Microwave for 30 more seconds and stir. Mixture should be the texture of scrambled eggs. Microwave longer, in 10-second increments, if eggs are not fully cooked.

4 Eat at once.

COOK'S NOTE: *Actual cooking time is about 2 minutes. Wash fork between stirs to reduce the possibility of eating raw egg. Make sure all ingredients are diced finely. Instead of the Turkey Sausage, dice Make Your Own Bacon or Pork Sausage Patties (p. 197 or p. 208,* The Migraine Relief Plan*). Skip the meat to make this vegetarian. Try fresh chèvre instead of ricotta. Use ½ cup of Breakfast Hash (p. 38) instead of the potatoes and peppers. If you're worried about the egg breaking in transit, crack it into the container before packing it for work. Use 2 eggs for a heartier breakfast; increase cooking time accordingly. Add a tablespoon of finely minced fresh herbs if you have them.*

PER SERVING (with whole-milk ricotta and store-bought turkey sausage; sodium will be lower if using Plan sausage):
21g protein, 9g carbohydrates, 15g fat, 7g saturated fat, 297mg sodium, 441mg potassium, 2g fiber

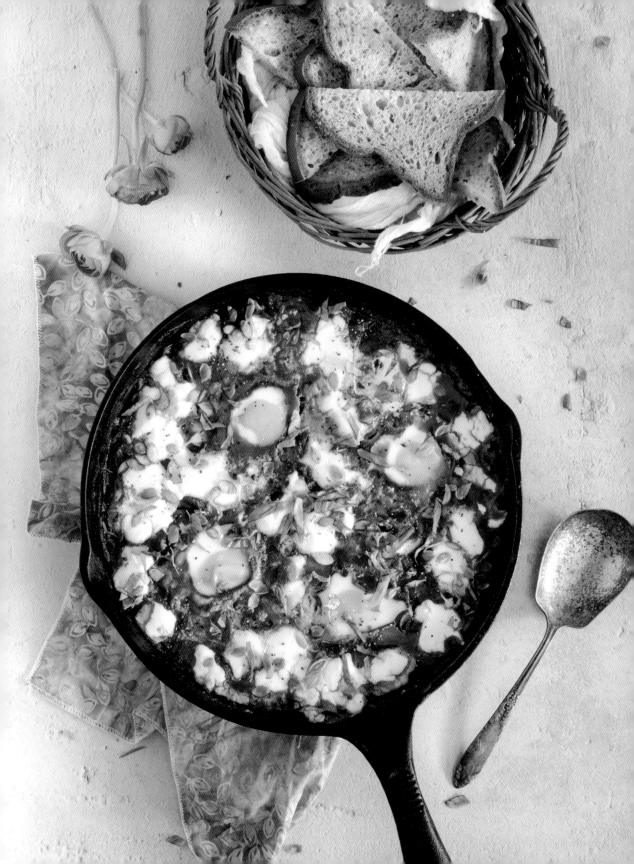

Tuscan Eggs

I love this dish served on top of gluten-free toast. This is a cross between two recipes from Tuscany: *uova alla Fiorentina* (eggs cooked with spinach but no tomato) and *uova al pomodoro* (eggs cooked in tomato but no spinach). It's definitely a weekend recipe, as it takes a little time to prepare.

Makes 4 servings

Prep time: 15 minutes
Cooking time: 40–45 minutes
Passive time: N/A

Budget friendly: Moderate

3 cups (700g) chunky no-salt-added tomato sauce, store-bought or Chunky Tomato Sauce (p. 188)

3 roasted red bell peppers, cut into strips or chunks

¾ cup (85g) frozen artichoke hearts

6 ounces (170g) fresh baby spinach or other dark, hearty greens, roughly chopped

½ teaspoon freshly ground black pepper

4 eggs

8 ounces (225g) ricotta cheese (omit to make the recipe dairy-free)

¼ cup (75g) raw pumpkin seeds

1 handful fresh basil leaves, slivered

1 Preheat the oven to 375°F (190°C).

2 In a large (12-inch [30cm]) oven-proof skillet, start heating the tomato sauce over medium heat. Stir in the vegetables as you finish prepping them: roasted bell peppers, artichoke hearts, spinach, or other greens.

3 Cover and cook until the greens wilt, about 10 minutes. Add the black pepper and stir everything gently to mix well.

4 Make 4 small wells in the top of the tomato mixture and crack an egg into each well.

5 Evenly distribute the ricotta cheese in large spoonfuls, then sprinkle with the pumpkin seeds. Turn off the burner and move the skillet to the oven.

6 Bake uncovered for 20 to 25 minutes, until the eggs are cooked, the sauce is bubbly, and the pumpkin seeds are golden brown.

7 Garnish with slivers of fresh basil and serve over polenta or gluten-free toast.

COOK'S NOTE: *Any no-salt-added tomato sauce or passata can be substituted for chunky tomato sauce without salt. Follow the method on page 32 to roast bell peppers, or use jarred roasted bell peppers, rinsed and drained.*

PER SERVING (with whole-milk ricotta cheese):
19g protein, 21g carbohydrates, 16g fat, 5g saturated fat, 276mg sodium, 603mg potassium, 6g fiber

Eggs Benedict

This decadent dish is probably my favorite to order when I go out for breakfast. Be sure to ask the restaurant if their hollandaise was prepared that morning. Undercooked eggs are often responsible for food poisoning (salmonella). If they can't guarantee it's fresh, skip it and make this special treat at home. Traditionally, Eggs Benedict made with spinach is called Eggs Florentine.

Makes 4 servings

Prep time: 30 minutes
Cooking time: 5 minutes
Passive time: N/A

Budget friendly: Very

8 ounces (225g) chopped spinach, kale, or other greens

4 pieces low-sodium gluten-free bread, toasted, or 4 slices polenta, grilled

4 eggs

3 egg yolks

1 tablespoon white vinegar

Pinch white pepper

½ cup (4 ounces/115g) butter, melted

COOK'S NOTE: *Refrigerate any leftover hollandaise immediately. Reheat and mix with leftover greens to use as a sauce over pasta or rice, or as a filling for Crepes (p. 200,* The Migraine Relief Plan*). Reheat hollandaise in a heat-proof container in the steamer over boiling water. Whisk before serving. It's not as good eaten later, but it is still yummy. Because the eggs in the sauce are not thoroughly cooked, it's safest to use pasteurized eggs if you can find them.*

1 Fill a large pan with 2 cups of tap water; place a steamer basket on top. Bring the water to a boil, then turn down the heat to simmer.

2 Add the greens to the steamer basket. Cover and steam until the greens are soft but still bright, approximately 3 to 5 minutes. Set greens aside in a bowl to keep warm. Return the steamer basket to the pan.

3 Set 4 sprayed or oiled ceramic ramekins in the steamer basket.

4 Toast the bread or grill the polenta while the ramekins are heating.

5 Crack the eggs into the ramekins, cover, and cook 4 minutes or until the egg whites are set but the yolks are still soft.

6 While the whole eggs are poaching, put the 3 egg yolks, vinegar, and white pepper in a blender. Start the blender on low, then turn up quickly to high. Immediately begin drizzling in the melted butter in a thin, steady stream. This should take about 30 seconds. The sauce should be fully thickened once the last of the butter is poured in. If not, blend 5 seconds longer until smooth. Don't over-blend, or the sauce may separate. You can also use an immersion blender to make the sauce.

7 Press the greens between a regular spoon and a slotted spoon to squeeze out excess moisture.

8 Place toast or polenta on a plate and top with one spoonful of greens and a poached egg. Pour sauce over greens and toast and serve immediately. Use leftover sauce within 3 days.

SERVING SUGGESTIONS: Add a side of Breakfast Hash (p. 38) to balance out the richness of this dish.

PER SERVING (with Trader Joe's Gluten-Free Multigrain Brown Rice Bread and unsalted butter):
12g protein, 23g carbohydrates, 34g fat, 17g saturated fat, 197mg sodium, 399mg potassium, 2g fiber

Strata

I have made this for so many brunches and holidays I've lost count. A perk of this recipe is how much you can vary it: with or without meat, with or without cheese, gluten-free for you, another pan with regular bread for guests. Make this up to one day ahead, then bake for an hour while you do other things.

Makes 12 servings

Prep time: 20 minutes
Cooking time: 60 minutes
Passive time: Overnight
                refrigeration
                plus 15 minutes
                to cool

Budget friendly: Very

6 eggs

¾ cup (180mL) whole or coconut milk

8 ounces (170g) ricotta cheese (omit for dairy-free version)

¼ teaspoon freshly ground black pepper

6 slices low-sodium gluten-free bread

8 ounces (225g) Turkey Sausage Patties (p. 51), cooked and crumbled (optional)

10 ounces (285g) frozen chopped broccoli, thawed and squeezed dry

1 In a large bowl, whisk the eggs, milk, ricotta if using, and pepper until blended.

2 Spray a 9 × 13-inch (23 x 33cm) baking dish with cooking spray, or lightly oil with coconut oil.

3 Cut the bread into cubes.

4 Add the bread cubes, meat, and broccoli in the dish in layers, evenly distributing the ingredients.

5 Pour the egg-milk mixture over it.

6 Cover with foil and refrigerate overnight.

7 In the morning, preheat the oven to 350°F (180°C). Pull the strata out of the refrigerator so it can begin coming to room temperature while the oven is preheating.

8 Bake strata uncovered for one hour until risen, puffed, and nicely browned.

9 Let cool about 15 minutes before cutting.

COOK'S NOTE: *Sautéed sliced mushrooms, thawed spinach (squeeze it dry before using), and/or sautéed sliced zucchini can be substituted for the broccoli. If you cannot find ricotta, cottage cheese is a good substitute, but blend it with the eggs and milk to smooth it out before Step 5.*

PER SERVING (without sausage, with whole milk and Trader Joe's Gluten-Free Multigrain Brown Rice Bread):
8g protein, 13g carbohydrates, 7g fat, 3g saturated fat, 105mg sodium, 151mg potassium, 1g fiber

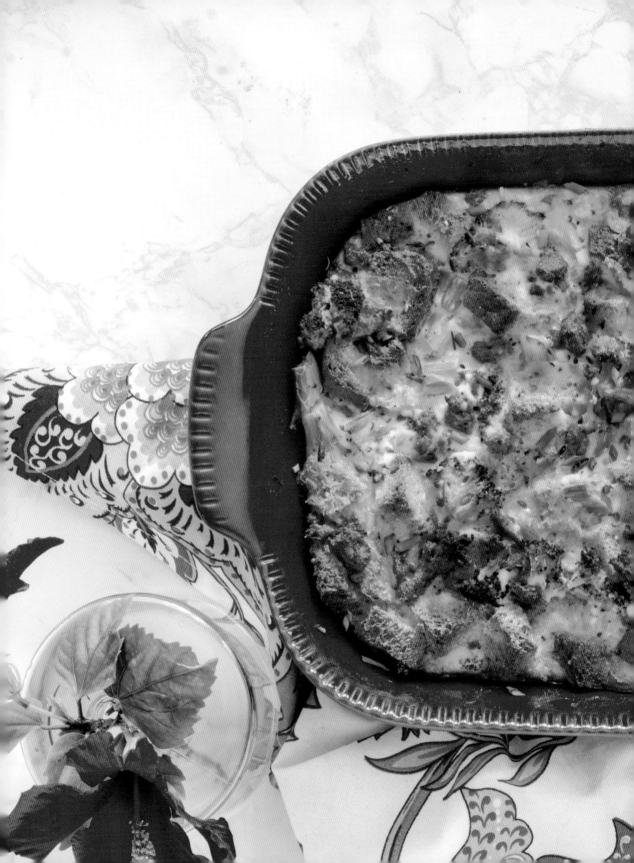

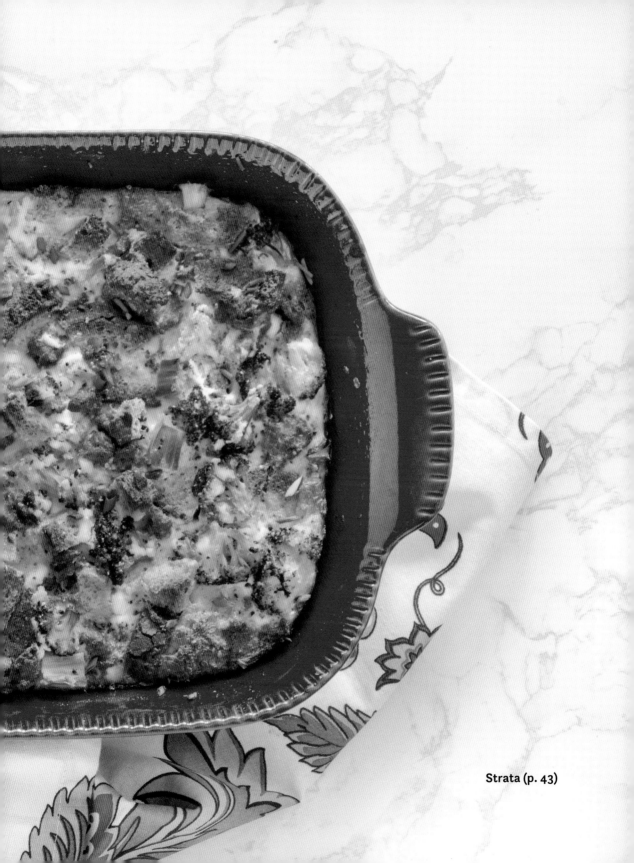

Strata (p. 43)

Pumpkin-Spice Waffles

I have always preferred waffles to pancakes, possibly because my mother was always in a hurry and her pancakes were often raw in the middle. Waffles were a special treat. I love how the melting butter pools inside the ridges. A seasonal take on one of my favorite breakfast foods, these are perfect for a chilly fall morning, but you can make them any time of year.

Makes 6–7 small square waffles

Prep time: 10 minutes
Cooking time: 20–25 minutes
Passive time: 5 minutes

Budget friendly: Very

1 tablespoon ground flax seeds or 1 egg

¾–1½ cups (180–360mL) whole, 2%, hemp, or coconut milk

¾ cup (185g) pumpkin puree, unsweetened

1½ teaspoons vanilla extract

1½ teaspoons baking powder

1½ teaspoons cinnamon

1 teaspoon ground ginger

1 teaspoon ground nutmeg

2 tablespoons cornmeal

1½ cups (145g) gluten-free flour such as Bob's Red Mill 1-to-1 Baking Flour or my Gluten-Free Flour Blend (p. 203)

Butter for serving

1 Preheat the waffle maker.

2 If using egg, add to blender. If using ground flax seeds as your egg replacer, add to blender with 2 tablespoons of filtered water and let sit five minutes.

3 Put the next seven ingredients into the blender (milk through nutmeg) and pulse a few times until well blended.

4 Add the cornmeal and pulse, then add the flour and pulse until just mixed. Batter will thicken as it stands. Add more milk as needed to maintain a pourable consistency.

5 Grease the waffle iron with oil or cooking spray and follow the manufacturer's instructions for filling and cooking the waffles. Make sure to spray or oil the iron between each one.

6 Serve hot with butter and a sprinkle of freshly grated nutmeg.

COOK'S NOTE: *Unsweetened applesauce can be substituted for the pumpkin puree.*

PER SERVING (with egg and hemp milk): 4g protein, 26g carbohydrates, 3g fat, 0g saturated fat, 149mg sodium, 27mg potassium, 2g fiber

"I think of resilience as this balance about where your feeling of control lies. Do you believe things happen to you, or do you believe you do things in the world? You can do something about your migraine. You can make those lifestyle changes, see the doctors, get treatments, do things that will help. Any time I'm not feeling resilient, it's when I have fallen to one side or another of that balance."

HART SHAFER, THERASPECS FOUNDER AND CEO

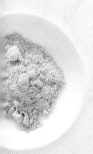
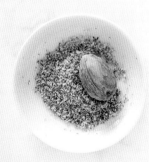
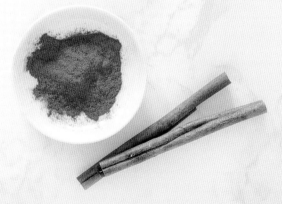

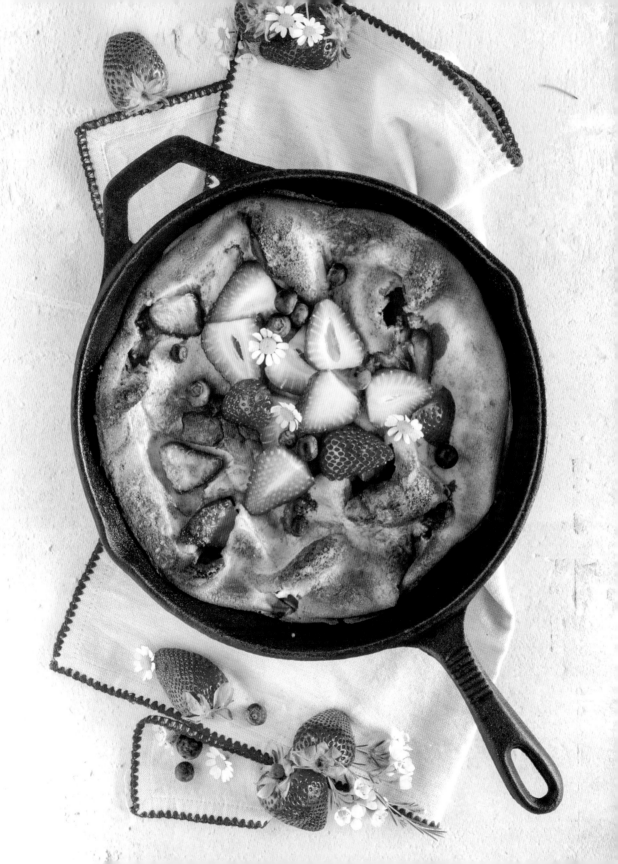

Dutch Baby Pancake

I love making puffy Dutch babies for a special brunch, especially on holiday weekends. I decided to make these grain-free for those folks who limit their grain intake. I think you'll find them surprisingly hearty. When topped with fresh fruit, they're elegant and loaded with healthy decadence.

Makes 2 servings

Prep time: 15 minutes
Cooking time: 25 minutes
Passive time: N/A

Budget friendly: Moderate

¼ cup (33g) sunflower seeds

¼ cup (28g) coconut flour

¼ cup (30g) tapioca flour

Stevia to equal 6 teaspoons sugar, divided

¾ cup (180mL) light coconut milk

1 teaspoon vanilla extract

3 eggs

2 tablespoons filtered water

1 cup strawberries, hulled and sliced

1 teaspoon cinnamon

1 tablespoon (15g) butter or coconut oil

1 Place a cast-iron or heat-proof skillet on the center rack of the oven.

2 Preheat oven to 450°F (230°C).

3 In a blender, grind the sunflower seeds to a fine powder. Use a butter knife to loosen seeds at the base of the blade.

4 Add the coconut flour, tapioca flour, and stevia to equal 4 teaspoons sugar and blend until mixed.

5 Add the coconut milk, vanilla extract, eggs, and water. Pulse until well blended.

6 Toss the strawberries with the cinnamon and remaining stevia and set aside.

7 When the oven comes to temperature, remove the pan using hot pads and set it on the stove. Add butter or coconut oil, swirling carefully to melt and completely coat the pan, including up the sides.

8 Pour in the strawberry mixture and shake the pan. Toss to coat the fruit with butter.

9 Pour the batter over the fruit and bake in the oven for 25 minutes, or until puffed and golden.

COOK'S NOTE: *Tapioca flour is the same thing as tapioca starch.*

SERVING SUGGESTIONS: Serve with butter or topped with Coconut Whipped Cream (p. 254, *The Migraine Relief Plan*), Berry Sauce (p. 250, *The Migraine Relief Plan*), or Vanilla Ricotta Cream (p. 263, *The Migraine Relief Plan*).

PER SERVING (with unsalted butter):
16g protein, 34g carbohydrates, 26g fat, 9g saturated fat, 139mg sodium, 383mg potassium, 11g fiber

Tex-Mex Migas

My mom, who grew up during the Depression, taught me to never waste food. But what to do with those leftover tortilla chip crumbs? Use them to make a Tex-Mex version of migas, which means "crumbs" in Spanish. Is it possible I hoard chips and salsa to make this? Yes.

Makes 2 servings

Prep time:	5 minutes
Cooking time:	10 minutes
Passive time:	N/A

Budget friendly: Very

1 cup (50g) no-salt-added tortilla chip pieces

1 tablespoon extra-virgin olive oil, ghee, or coconut oil

1 cup (250mL) low-sodium salsa (see Cook's Note)

2 eggs

1–2 tablespoons half and half, heavy cream, or coconut milk

¼ teaspoon freshly ground black pepper

1 In a plastic bag or bowl, crunch the tortilla crumbs to the size of bread crumbs.

2 Heat a nonstick frying pan over medium heat. Add the olive oil and tilt pan to coat.

3 Sauté the tortilla crumbs until golden brown.

4 Pour the salsa over the crumbs and continue to cook until they start to soften.

5 In a small bowl, whisk the eggs with the half and half and the pepper.

6 Pour the eggs into the pan and continue to cook and stir until the eggs are nearly set.

7 Flip in portions until everything is cooked through.

COOK'S NOTE: *Instead of store-bought salsa, use Salsa Fresca (p. 190) or Salsa Verde (p. 274,* The Migraine Relief Plan*).*

SERVING SUGGESTIONS: Add a side of Breakfast Hash (p. 38) and Make Your Own Bacon (p. 197, *The Migraine Relief Plan*).

PER SERVING: 9g protein, 33g carbohydrates, 18g fat, 9g saturated fat, 158mg sodium, 84mg potassium, 2g fiber

Turkey Sausage Patties

One of the challenges of eating a low-sodium diet is that packaged breakfast meats are off the table. But with this recipe, you can make your own turkey or chicken sausage patties. I love the flavors of sage, garlic, and thyme, which remind me a bit of Thanksgiving, and the richness added by the smoked paprika.

Makes 13 patties

Prep time: 10 minutes
Cooking time: 10 minutes
Passive time: N/A

Budget friendly: Very

1 ¼ pound (570g) ground turkey (93% lean) or ground chicken, defrosted overnight if frozen

1½ teaspoons dried sage

1½ teaspoons garlic powder

1 teaspoon dried thyme

1 teaspoon smoked paprika

½ teaspoon black pepper

½ teaspoon cream of tartar (optional)

¼ teaspoon cayenne pepper (optional)

2 tablespoons extra-virgin olive oil, divided

1 Place the turkey or chicken in a large bowl. Mix all the spices together in a small bowl until they are well combined.

2 With your hands, evenly incorporate the spice mixture and 1 tablespoon of the olive oil with the meat.

3 Shape into 13 equal-sized patties, each about 2 inches (5cm) in diameter. I use a small ice cream scoop, then flatten them with my hand. Place on a plate until ready to fry.

4 Heat a large griddle or nonstick frying pan over medium heat. Add the remaining olive oil.

5 Pan fry until no longer pink in the center, about 3 to 5 minutes on each side.

COOK'S NOTE: *Cream of tartar makes the patties more tender, but some people are sensitive to it. Skip the cayenne if making for those sensitive to spicy foods. Roasted garlic powder adds another layer of savory, rich flavor. My preferred ice cream scoop is Size 24 (1.5 fluid ounces [44mL]). If you plan to freeze leftovers, allow patties to cool before placing in freezer-safe containers.*

SERVING SUGGESTIONS: These pair beautifully with Breakfast Hash (p. 38) and an over-easy egg. Use as a sausage crumble in Quickie Microwave Egg Scramble (p. 39), Frittata (p. 280, *The Migraine Relief Plan*), Pizza (p. 284, *The Migraine Relief Plan*), Quiche (p. 285, *The Migraine Relief Plan*), or Rice Bowl (p. 286, *The Migraine Relief Plan*).

PER SERVING: 10g protein, 0g carbohydrates, 3g fat, 0g saturated fat, 0mg sodium, 0mg potassium, 0g fiber

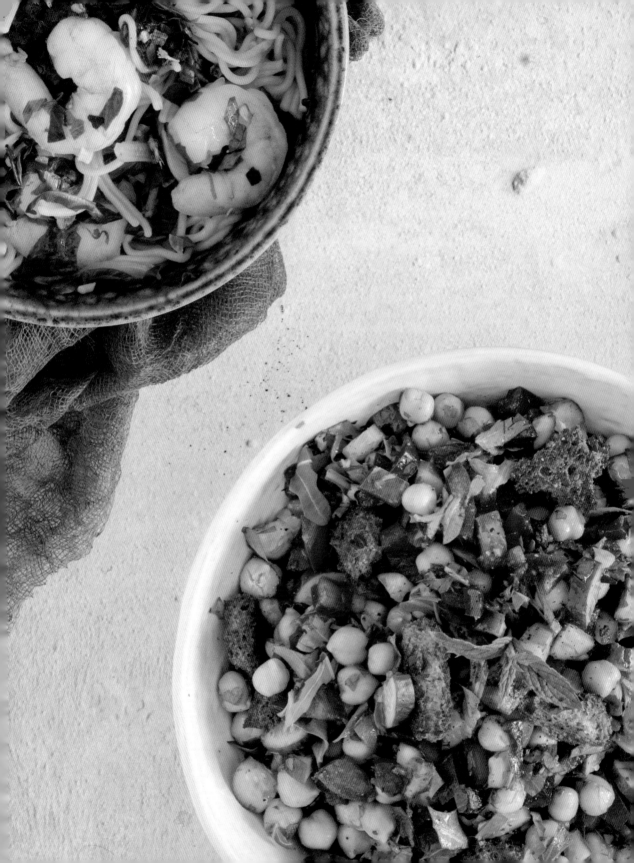

Salads and Light Meals

On migraine attack days, if I'm hungry at all, I usually want to eat something light. I've included a variety of salad ideas that might bring new flavors into your life, two light burger options, and a ramen bowl that's quick to make and easy to digest when I'm feeling nauseated. I also invented a chorizo substitute made from quinoa for vegetarians who love soy chorizo but might find it to be a trigger.

Mango Chicken Salad

I love fruity salsas, especially mango salsa. Since mango is one of the few tropical fruits on the Plan, I was inspired to try combining the flavors from a mango salsa—red bell pepper, jalapeño, and hot sauce—to create this fresh twist on a classic. Make this sweet and spicy chicken salad from leftover roasted chicken breast.

Makes 4 servings

Prep time: 10 minutes
Cooking time: N/A
Passive time: N/A

Budget friendly: Very

12 ounces (340g) cooked skinless chicken breast, diced

6 tablespoons mayonnaise, store-bought or my Egg-Free Mayonnaise (p. 194) or Olive Oil Mayonnaise (p. 195)

1 mango, diced

1 red bell pepper, diced

½ cup (60g) toasted pumpkin seeds

1 jalapeño, minced (or to taste)

Dash Hot Sauce (p. 196)

1 Add all the ingredients to a large bowl and stir until well-combined.

COOK'S NOTE: *Using one of my homemade mayo recipes controls the sodium in this recipe. In place of Hot Sauce, try a dash of Chile Pepper Sauce (p. 267, The Migraine Relief Plan).*

 If limes are not a trigger for you, a squeeze of lime juice makes this sing.

SERVING SUGGESTIONS: Serve over a large bowl of spring mix or as an open-face sandwich on gluten-free toast.

PER SERVING (sodium and fat will be lower if made using leftover chicken breast from Roasted Chicken with Veggie Gravy [p. 134] and homemade mayo): 45g protein, 13g carbohydrates, 31g fat, 7g saturated fat, 204mg sodium, 373mg potassium, 3g fiber

"I've had to deal with a lot of implicit biases, especially seeking care in the emergency room or urgent care setting. Black women in pain are just completely invisible. It's like our pain doesn't exist at all. Lean into your own knowledge about yourself, your condition, what your treatment is, what has failed you in the past, and what has worked for you. Lean into that and don't settle for less than adequate treatment. You're a human being and you deserve better care, regardless of your race. Everybody deserves that."

JAIME MICHELE SANDERS, *THE MIGRAINE DIVA*

Curried Chicken Salad

Make this easy chicken salad with leftover roasted chicken breast and a few simple ingredients. While it's delicious served as a sandwich with gluten-free toast, I love pairing it with tender butter lettuce, which picks up the sweetness of the apple and crunch of the celery. As long as you keep it well-chilled, it's a terrific on-the-go lunch or picnic food.

Makes 4 servings

Prep time: 10 minutes
Cooking time: N/A
Passive time: N/A

Budget friendly: Very

1½ teaspoons no-salt-added curry powder, mild or medium-heat

6 tablespoons mayonnaise, store-bought or my Egg-Free Mayonnaise (p. 194) or Olive Oil Mayonnaise (p. 195)

12 ounces (340g) cooked skinless chicken breast, diced

1 apple, cored and diced

1 stalk celery, diced

½ cup toasted sunflower seeds

1 Whisk the curry powder into the mayo in a large serving or storage bowl.

2 Add the other ingredients and mix well.

COOK'S NOTE: *Try making this with leftover Roasted Chicken (p. 134) or Lazy Chicken (p. 90). You can substitute red seedless grapes (cut in half) for the apple. See note on page 18 if you have questions about curry powder.*

SERVING SUGGESTIONS: Serve over lettuce, fresh spinach, or baby arugula. For picnics, serve with these other travel-friendly, chilled dishes: Provençal Chickpea Salad (p. 218, *The Migraine Relief Plan*), Three Bean and Potato Salad (p. 222, *The Migraine Relief Plan*), Berry Trifle (p. 253, *The Migraine Relief Plan*), Cucumber-Basil Water (p. 258, *The Migraine Relief Plan*), Strawberry-Mint Water (p. 259, *The Migraine Relief Plan*).

PER SERVING: 26g protein, 11g carbohydrates, 26g fat, 3g saturated fat, 145mg sodium, 96mg potassium, 4g fiber

"I like to ask: What are my strengths? What are my superpowers? What superpower can I use in a creative way to make my life different? You don't have to start with a really big step. For me, I didn't jump in and start flying aerobatics on the first day. The first day I just drove to the airport and tried not to throw up."

DR. CECILIA ARAGON, AUTHOR OF
FLYING FREE: MY VICTORY OVER
FEAR TO BECOME THE FIRST LATINA
PILOT ON THE US AEROBATIC TEAM

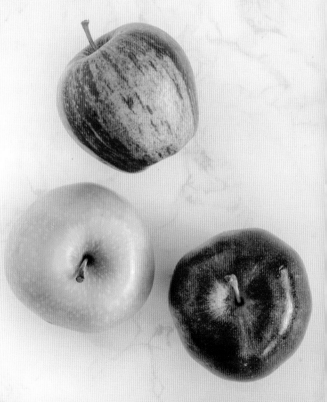

Grilled Chicken Caesar Salad

A true Caesar salad includes parmesan and anchovies. I use dry mustard and smoked paprika to create a rich, complex garlicky dressing instead. You won't miss the cheese. Grilling all the components adds layers of smoky flavor. If you've never had grilled romaine, try it once just for me.

**Makes 2 servings,
with extra dressing**

Prep time: 15 minutes
Cooking time: 12–15 minutes
Passive time: N/A

Budget friendly: Very

2 pieces low-sodium gluten-free bread

¼ cup (60mL) extra-virgin olive oil, plus more for brushing

1 clove garlic, cut in half

24 fresh basil leaves, divided

2 tablespoons filtered water

1 tablespoon mayonnaise, store-bought or my Egg-Free Mayonnaise (p. 194) or Olive Oil Mayonnaise (p. 195)

2 teaspoons white vinegar

¼ teaspoon dry mustard

1 chicken breast, boneless and skinless, butterflied and pounded thin (see Cook's Note)

1 teaspoon smoked paprika

1 teaspoon black pepper

1 large head romaine lettuce

 If they are not a trigger for you, substitute lemon juice or white balsamic vinegar for the white vinegar.

1 Prepare the bread by lightly brushing with olive oil and rubbing with the cut garlic.

2 Make the dressing. Add the garlic clove, the olive oil, half the basil, the water, the mayonnaise, the vinegar, and the mustard to a blender and blend until smooth. Set aside.

3 Heat a grill or grill pan to medium-high.

4 Season both sides of the chicken with the smoked paprika and black pepper.

5 Grill the chicken 4 minutes per side, until cooked through but still juicy. Place on a clean cutting board to rest.

6 Grill the bread 2 to 4 minutes per side, then use a serrated knife to cube into croutons.

7 Slice the romaine lettuce in half lengthwise, leaving the core intact. Grill for two minutes per side.

8 Slice the grilled romaine crosswise into thin ribbons, discarding the core, and divide between two plates. Slice the chicken and add on top. Sprinkle the croutons and reserved basil leaves over the salad. Drizzle with 1 tablespoon dressing per salad. Serve at once.

COOK'S NOTE: *To butterfly the chicken breast: Place chicken on a piece of heavy plastic wrap on your cutting board. With your knife parallel to the cutting board, slice the chicken along one of its longer edges, starting at the thickest point. Do not cut all the way through to the other side; stop about 2/3 of the way across. Fold open the chicken breast, as if opening a book, to lay flat. Cover with another piece of plastic wrap. Pound the entire piece with a meat mallet, rolling pin, or a heavy cast-iron pan until the meat is all the same thickness, about ½-inch (1.25 cm) thick. Omit bread for grain-free version.*

PER SERVING (salad with 1 tablespoon dressing):
42g protein, 29g carbohydrates, 8g fat, 1g saturated fat, 205mg sodium, 773mg potassium, 8g fiber

Fattoush Salad

This Middle Eastern salad normally uses leftover pita bread that's fried for a crispy texture. Instead, I bake it into crunchy pieces, which contrast with the bright, fresh, chopped herbs and vegetables. Dried sumac is optional but adds authentic flavor.

Makes 6 servings

Prep time: 20 minutes
Cooking time: 7 minutes
Passive time: 15 minutes

Budget friendly: Very

4 tablespoons (60mL) extra-virgin olive oil

2 ½ teaspoons white vinegar

¾ teaspoon ground sumac (optional), divided

¼ teaspoon ground cumin

⅛ teaspoon dry mustard

1⅛ teaspoons garlic powder or granules, divided

⅛ teaspoon white pepper

2 green onions, thinly sliced

2 slices gluten-free bread, gluten-free pita, or 1 gluten-free frozen pizza crust, thawed

Cooking spray or olive oil for spraying on bread pieces

1 cup (225g) tomatoes, chopped

1 cup (225g) English or Persian cucumbers, sliced

½ cup (115g) diced red bell peppers

½ cup (115g) chopped fresh Italian parsley

½ cup (115g) chopped fresh mint leaves

½ cup (115g) chopped arugula (rocket)

1 (15-ounce [425g]) can no-salt-added black-eyed peas or garbanzo beans, rinsed and drained

1 Preheat the oven to 400°F (200°C).

2 Combine the olive oil, the vinegar, ½ teaspoon of the sumac (if using), the cumin, the dry mustard, ⅛ teaspoon of the garlic powder, and the white pepper in a jar with a tightly fitting lid. Shake well to combine.

3 Put the green onions in a bowl of very cold water and soak for 10 minutes to remove the sharp taste. Drain thoroughly and pat dry with a kitchen or paper towel.

4 Meanwhile, tear the bread into irregular pieces. Arrange in a single layer on a baking sheet lined with parchment paper. Spray lightly with cooking oil spray or brush with olive oil. Sprinkle lightly with the remaining 1 teaspoon garlic powder.

5 Bake for 7 minutes, stirring after 4 minutes. Cool completely.

6 Combine the tomatoes and last 6 ingredients in a large bowl.

7 Add the toasted bread to the bowl, reserving 2 handfuls for topping. Add the dressing and toss well to coat.

8 Top evenly with reserved toasted bread and sprinkle with the remaining ¼ teaspoon sumac (if using).

COOK'S NOTE: *Look for gluten-free pita bread, gluten-free flatbread, or gluten-free pizza crust in the frozen section of large grocery stores. Trader Joe's Multigrain Brown Rice Gluten-Free Bread is a good option for low-sodium diets.*

SERVING SUGGESTIONS: Top with leftover grilled chicken to make a complete meal.

PER SERVING (Using Trader Joe's Multigrain Brown Rice Gluten-Free Bread and canned black-eyed peas): 5g protein, 19g carbohydrates, 10g fat, 2g saturated fat, 229mg sodium, 137mg potassium, 3g fiber

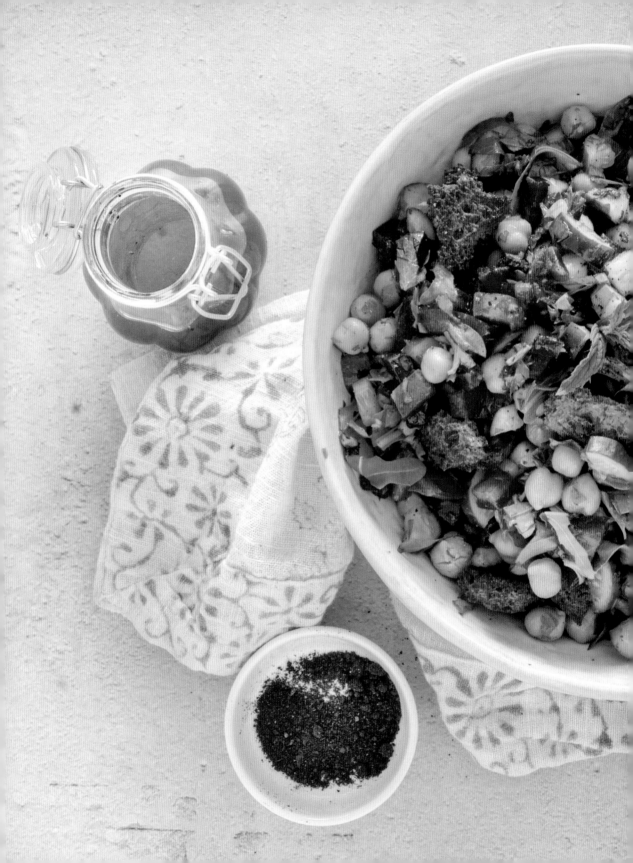

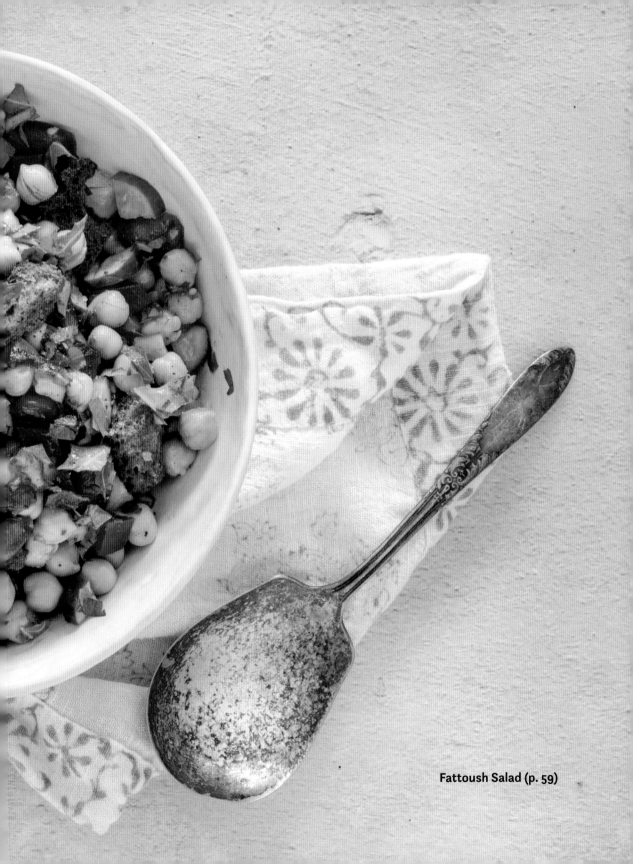

Fattoush Salad (p. 59)

Tuna-Rice Salad

I grew up eating canned tuna, with no idea of the health benefits of fatty fish. I first made this salad with leftover brown rice on a hot summer evening when I was living with a dear friend in Chicago. We realized it had all the flavors of a tuna-salad sandwich without the bread, and the rainbow of vegetables provides color, nutrients, and crunch.

Makes 4 servings

Prep time: 10 minutes
Cooking time: N/A
Passive time: N/A

Budget friendly: Very

1 cup (190g) cooked short-grain brown rice

1 (5-ounce [142g]) can no-salt-added albacore tuna, drained

2 small cucumbers, peeled and diced

1 carrot, grated

¼ red bell pepper, diced

¼ cup (58g) mayonnaise, store-bought or Egg-Free Mayonnaise (p. 194) or Olive Oil Mayonnaise (p. 195)

½ teaspoon freshly ground black pepper

1 Mix everything together and serve over greens.

COOK'S NOTE: *I prefer the texture and nuttiness of short-grain brown rice in this salad, but you can substitute any cooked brown rice. Substitute celery if you don't have cucumbers. Using homemade mayonnaise reduces the sodium considerably.*

"Resilience is about learning to bend and adapt and flow with what life brings, even when it's unexpected, or even when it's not what we want. Letting go of that need or desire to control everything that happens in my life has been key."

DANIELLE SIMONE BRAND, AUTHOR OF *WEED MOM: THE CANNA-CURIOUS WOMAN'S GUIDE TO HEALTHIER RELAXATION, HAPPIER PARENTING, AND CHILLING TF OUT*

PER SERVING (with store-bought mayo):
10g protein, 14g carbohydrates, 11g fat, 2g saturated fat, 115mg sodium, 128mg potassium, 2g fiber

Honey-Mustard Salmon Salad

Canned salmon is a convenient source of protein, calcium, and omega-3s. But for me, the tinny taste can be a turn-off. In this recipe, the sweetness of raw honey and the sharpness of dry mustard transform this versatile pantry staple into something surprising, masking any canned flavor. It's also a quick, inexpensive way to get a serving of fatty fish into my diet.

Makes 2 servings

Prep time: 5 minutes
Cooking time: N/A
Passive time: N/A

Budget friendly: Very

2–3 tablespoons mayonnaise, store-bought or my Egg-Free Mayonnaise (p. 194) or Olive Oil Mayonnaise (p. 195)

1–2 teaspoons honey

½ teaspoon dry mustard

¼ teaspoon freshly ground black pepper

1 (6-ounce [170g]) can no-salt-added wild-caught Alaskan pink salmon, drained

1 In a medium bowl, mix together the mayonnaise, honey, dry mustard, and black pepper.

2 Add the salmon and stir well.

COOK'S NOTE: *Use Olive Oil Mayonnaise (p. 195) or Egg-Free Mayonnaise (p. 194) to make this very low in sodium. Some testers preferred less mayonnaise and less honey, and one added chopped celery. Adjust ingredients to suit your taste. Using dry mustard provides mustard flavor without the sodium or fermentation of jarred mustard. If you can afford it, Manuka honey from New Zealand contains much higher levels of methylglyoxal, believed to provide antibacterial, antiviral, anti-inflammatory, and antioxidant benefits.*

SERVING SUGGESTIONS: Serve a scoop on top of a big salad of greens and chopped raw vegetables, or as a sandwich with lettuce on toasted gluten-free bread.

PER SERVING (made with 3 tablespoons Trader Joe's Organic Mayonnaise; sodium level will be much lower with homemade mayo):
20g protein, 6g carbohydrates, 18g fat, 2g saturated fat, 218mg sodium, 4mg potassium, 0g fiber

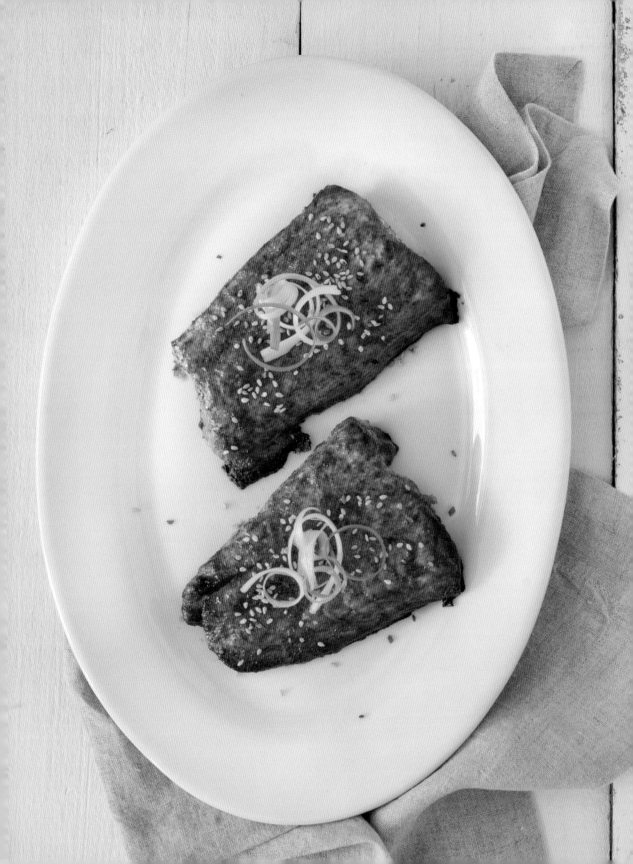

Grilled Salmon, Two Glazes

A recent study showed promising results on the impact of omega-3 fatty acids, like those found in salmon, in reducing migraine attack frequency and intensity (see endnote 7 on page 216). My first thought when I read that study was to take more omega-3 supplements, but I know from my public health training that it's always preferable to eat whole foods versus taking a supplement, as the food provides additional nutrients and flavor. I've given you two options to create a quick, easy glaze for grilled salmon.

Makes 2 servings

Prep time: 5 minutes
Cooking time: 5 minutes
Passive time: N/A

Budget friendly: Moderate

Honey Sesame Ginger Glaze:

1 teaspoon honey, warmed

1 teaspoon toasted dark sesame oil

¼ teaspoon freshly grated ginger root

Garnish: ½ teaspoon sesame seeds

Smoky Maple Glaze:

1 teaspoon pure maple syrup

1 teaspoon extra-virgin olive oil

1 teaspoon smoked paprika

8 ounces (225g) wild-caught Alaskan salmon steaks or fillets, thawed if frozen, cut into 2 equal portions

1 Prepare glaze of choice.

2 Place the salmon on a pan lined with a sheet of heavy aluminum foil. Brush or spoon glaze over salmon.

3 Turn on grill or broiler. Grill or broil for 5 minutes or until fish is crispy on the edges and cooked through in the thickest part. You can also bake the salmon at 400°F (200°C) for 12 to 18 minutes, just until the center is cooked through.

4 Garnish Honey Sesame Ginger salmon with the sesame seeds.

5 Serve immediately.

COOK'S NOTE: *If salmon is frozen, thaw overnight in the refrigerator. Cutting fish into portions allows it to cook faster and gives every piece lovely caramelized edges. Choose salmon pieces that are uniformly thick.*

SERVING SUGGESTIONS: Serve with Fattoush Salad (p. 59), Chipotle Sweet Potatoes (p. 112), Coconut-Curried Greens (p. 110), Lebanese Green Beans (p. 118), Chopped Salad (p. 287, *The Migraine Relief Plan*), Spicy Kale and Swiss Chard Sauté (p. 243, *The Migraine Relief Plan*), Wild Rice and Carrots (p. 246, *The Migraine Relief Plan*).

PER SERVING: 22g protein, 2g carbohydrates, 5g fat, 1g saturated fat, 75mg sodium, 3mg potassium, 0g fiber

Quinrizo Taco Salad

If you love the flavors of restaurant taco salads, here's a healthy twist. It all starts with Quinrizo, my vegetarian chorizo substitute made from quinoa. Add crisp romaine, bright vegetables, beans for protein, and chips for crunch. Top with my spicy, creamy dressing.

Makes 8 servings

Prep time: 30 minutes
Cooking time: 35 minutes
Passive time: 30 minutes–
                24 hours

Budget friendly: Moderate

¼ cup (58g) mayonnaise, store-bought or my Egg-Free Mayonnaise (p. 194) or Olive Oil Mayonnaise (p. 195)

2 tablespoons Hot Sauce (p. 196) or to taste

2 tablespoons whole or coconut milk

½ teaspoon white vinegar

¼ teaspoon ground cumin

Quinrizo (recipe follows)

1 pint cherry tomatoes, chopped

1 yellow, red, or orange bell pepper, chopped

1 head romaine lettuce, shredded

1 (14.5-ounce [411g]) can no-salt-added pinto or kidney beans, rinsed and drained

4 green onions, thinly sliced

1 cup (50g) minced cilantro or fresh Italian parsley

8 ounces (28g) no-salt-added tortilla chips, crushed

1 Make the dressing by whisking together the first 5 ingredients (mayonnaise through cumin). Thin with filtered water to make a pourable dressing.

2 Place the next 7 ingredients (Quinrizo through cilantro) in a large serving bowl.

3 Pour dressing over the salad and toss to coat.

4 Add the chips right before serving.

COOK'S NOTE: *Sub Chile Pepper Sauce (p. 267, The Migraine Relief Plan) for Hot Sauce to make a milder dressing. If you can't find no-salt-added tortilla chips, toast corn tortillas until very crispy. If you won't be eating the entire salad, dress the servings individually so the lettuce doesn't get soggy. In recipes using only the white parts of the green onions, I save the green parts in the freezer to make Low-Sodium Chicken Broth (p. 136).*

PER SERVING: 10g protein, 43g carbohydrates, 17g fat, 2g saturated fat, 152mg sodium, 350mg potassium, 10g fiber

Quinrizo *(meat-free chorizo substitute)*

1 cup (180g) uncooked quinoa, any color, rinsed and drained

1 cup (237mL) low-sodium vegetable broth or Low-Sodium Chicken Broth (p. 136)

1 medium tomato, cored and quartered or ½ cup (115g) diced canned no-salt-added tomatoes, drained

6 green onions, white parts only

3 cloves garlic

1 tablespoon white vinegar

1 teaspoon ground cumin

1 teaspoon smoked paprika

1 teaspoon dried oregano

¾ teaspoon chipotle powder

2 tablespoons extra-virgin olive oil, divided

1 Bring the quinoa and broth to a boil in a medium saucepan with a lid. Turn the heat to low and cook, covered, for 15 minutes. Turn off the heat, leaving the pan on the burner. Let sit at least 10 minutes, then remove lid and fluff with a fork. Quinoa should be on the dry side.

2 Process the tomato, onions, garlic, vinegar, and spices in a food processor into a fairly smooth mixture with no large chunks. Pause once or twice to scrape down the sides.

3 Add the cooked, fluffed quinoa to a large mixing bowl, then add 1 tablespoon of the olive oil and stir until completely coated. Add the mixture from the food processor and mix completely. Cover and refrigerate at least 30 minutes, but preferably overnight, to infuse the quinoa with maximum flavor.

4 Heat the remaining 1 tablespoon olive oil in a large nonstick saucepan or cast-iron frying pan on medium heat, then add the quinoa mixture. Cook for 20 minutes, stirring every few minutes to keep it from sticking.

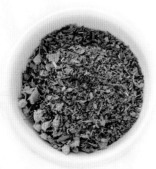
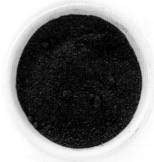
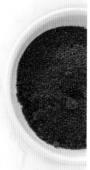

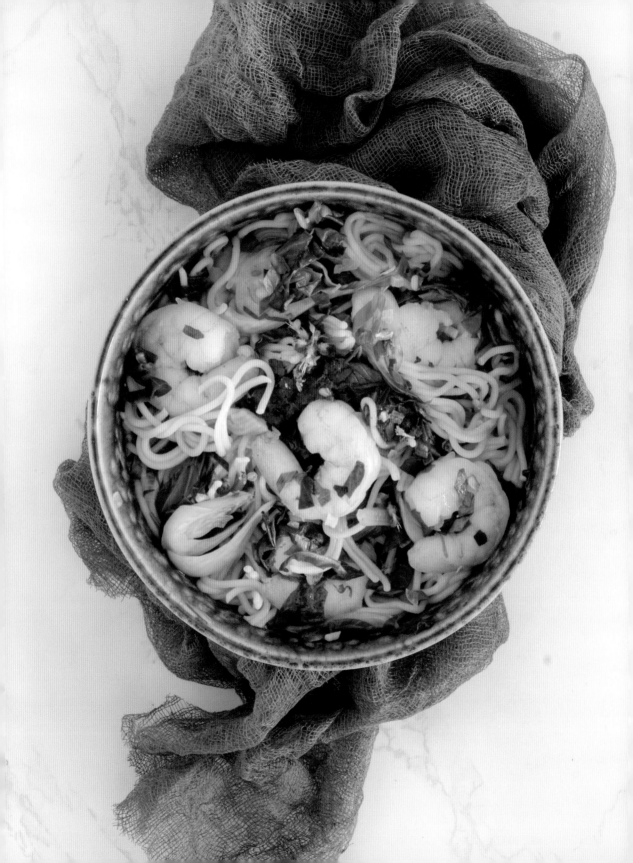

Quick and Easy Ramen

Who doesn't love ramen? Slurping noodles out of a generous bowl of broth, fishing out meat and vegetables along the way. But traditional ramen, made from wheat-based noodles and soy-enhanced broth, is full of potential migraine triggers for me. When I spotted rice-based ramen noodles in my grocery store, I had to try making my own Plan-friendly ramen at home. It completely satisfies my craving for this Japanese staple.

Makes 1 serving

Prep time: 5 minutes
Cooking time: 10 minutes
Passive time: N/A

Budget friendly: Very

2 cups(473mL) no-salt-added chicken or vegetable broth

1 green onion, thinly sliced

1 clove garlic, minced or pressed

1 shallot, minced (optional)

1 block (2 ½ ounces [70g]) rice-based ramen noodles

6 frozen shell-off shrimp or ½ cup (70g) cooked diced chicken

1 baby bok choy, thinly sliced

2 handfuls spinach, about 2 cups (60g), loosely packed

If coconut aminos are not a migraine trigger for you, add a splash.

1 Combine the broth, green onion, garlic, and shallot (if using) in a saucepan. Bring to a boil over medium-high heat. Turn down heat so it's not rapidly boiling, but a bubble breaks the surface here and there.

2 Add the noodles and stir with a fork to break them apart. Cook 3 to 4 minutes.

3 Drain the noodles and capture the broth. Place noodles into a serving bowl; return the broth to saucepan.

4 Stir the protein and greens into the broth. Cook for another 4 to 5 minutes until shrimp are pink (if using) or chicken is hot. Pour over the noodles and eat at once.

COOK'S NOTE: *The only brand of rice-based ramen noodles I have found is made by Lotus Foods, which can be ordered online. I tried 3 types of rice vermicelli in 2-ounce portions, all of which worked. Buckwheat soba noodles did not provide an appetizing result.*

SERVING SUGGESTIONS: Optional add-ins include 1 sliced hard-boiled egg, Hot Sauce (p. 196) to taste, up to 1 tablespoon grass-fed ghee, or 1 teaspoon garlic powder.

PER SERVING (1 Lotus Foods ramen cake, 3.5 ounces cooked chicken breast):
47g protein, 61g carbohydrates, 7g fat, 1g saturated fat, 314mg sodium, 1235mg potassium, 6g fiber

Mediterranean Tuna Burgers

I am lucky to have neighbors who fish off the coast of San Diego. When they brought me tuna steaks for the first time, I developed this recipe as an alternative to grilling the steaks plain. The bright herbs and olive oil bring out the flavor of the tuna, and I can imagine myself on a patio overlooking the Mediterranean Sea.

Makes 4 burgers

Prep time: 5 minutes
Cooking time: 6 minutes
Passive time: N/A

Budget friendly: Moderate

2 green onions, roughly chopped

3 cloves garlic

2 tablespoons fresh basil leaves, firmly packed

1 tablespoon fresh oregano leaves, or 1 teaspoon dried

1 pound (450g) tuna steaks, thawed if frozen, cut into large chunks

1–2 tablespoons extra-virgin olive oil

½ teaspoon freshly ground black pepper

⅛ teaspoon fine sea salt

1 Heat a grill, grill pan, or electric grill to medium-high heat.

2 Pulse the green onions, garlic, basil, and oregano in a food processor until finely chopped, stopping once to scrape down the sides.

3 Add the tuna. Pulse twice.

4 Add 1 tablespoon of the olive oil, the pepper, and the salt, and pulse a few more times until the tuna is just chopped and the mixture binds together. Add additional olive oil if the mixture seems too dry.

5 Form into four patties.

6 Oil the grill or grill pan and turn down to medium. If using a grill, cook over indirect heat.

7 Cook for 3 to 4 minutes on the first side. Watch the side of the meat; once the burger deepens in color halfway, it's time to flip. Flip and cook for 2 to 3 minutes more. Remove from heat and serve immediately.

COOK'S NOTE: *Frozen fish is best thawed in the refrigerator overnight to preserve its texture. If you don't have access to fresh herbs, use 1 tablespoon no-salt-added Italian seasoning in place of the fresh basil and fresh or dried oregano. I've swapped fresh mint for the basil and loved the results. You can use swordfish, mahi mahi, or salmon in this recipe as well. Burgers should be cooked through, not pink in the middle.*

SERVING SUGGESTIONS: Serve on gluten-free buns with a side salad. Substitute butter lettuce or Savoy cabbage leaves for the buns if you're following a low-carb diet.

PER 4-OUNCE BURGER (with 2 tablespoons olive oil):
28g protein, 2g carbohydrates, 8g fat, 1g saturated fat, 84mg sodium, 46mg potassium, 1g fiber

Veggie Burgers

After *The Migraine Relief Plan* came out, I had requests for more vegetarian recipes. This hearty veggie burger is inspired by one I enjoy at a San Diego restaurant called Station Tavern. The mild flavor of the chickpeas is amped up with carrots, mushrooms, leeks, and spices. While frozen veggie burgers are available, they're usually high in sodium and include onions, which are not Plan-friendly.

Makes 6 burgers

Prep time: 20 minutes
Cooking time: 25 minutes
Passive time: 30 minutes

Budget friendly: Very

1½ teaspoons ground flax seeds

2 tablespoons extra-virgin olive oil, divided

1 medium carrot (75g), diced (about ½ cup)

4 ounces cremini mushrooms, sliced

1 cup (90g) cleaned, thinly sliced leeks

1 tablespoon garlic powder or granulated garlic

1 teaspoon ground cumin

½ teaspoon freshly ground black pepper

¼ teaspoon red pepper flakes

1 slice low-sodium gluten-free bread, toasted

1 (15-ounce [425g]) can no-salt-added chickpeas, drained and rinsed, or 1¾ cups home-cooked chickpeas

1 Combine the ground flax seeds in a large bowl with 1 tablespoon filtered water.

2 Heat 1 tablespoon of the olive oil over medium heat in a large nonstick sauté pan until it shimmers. Swirl to coat evenly. Sauté the carrot, mushrooms, leeks, garlic powder, cumin, and black and red pepper for 7 to 8 minutes until golden brown. Remove from the heat.

3 Tear the toasted bread into pieces and add to a food processor. Pulse to make medium-size breadcrumbs. Transfer to the large bowl containing the flax seeds.

4 Pulse the cooked carrot mixture in the food processor until roughly chopped. Transfer to the large bowl.

5 Pulse half the chickpeas with the remaining 1 tablespoon olive oil in the food processor until fairly smooth. Transfer to the large bowl and stir well.

6 Pulse the remaining chickpeas 10 times, until roughly chopped. Transfer to the mixture in the large bowl.

7 Stir, mashing well, until the mixture forms a thick paste that can be shaped into burgers. Add water 1 teaspoon at a time if needed.

8 To make each burger, firmly pack the mixture into patties using an egg ring (or other tool; see Cook's Note) set on a baking sheet lined with parchment paper or on a silicone sheet. Repeat. Chill at least 30 minutes, up to overnight.

9 Grill or pan-fry the burgers over medium heat with a small amount of olive oil until golden brown, 6 minutes per side.

COOK'S NOTE: *If using frozen or pre-cleaned leeks, you'll need 1 cup sliced (90g). Form uniform patties using egg rings, a large ice cream scooper, a muffin-top pan, or canning lids. These patties are not as sturdy as meat-based burgers so be careful when turning them. These freeze well, uncooked. Cook 8 to 10 minutes per side if frozen.*

PER 3½-INCH BURGER (using Trader Joe's Gluten-Free Multigrain Brown Rice Bread):
6g protein, 17g carbohydrates, 6g fat, 1g saturated fat, 39mg sodium, 407mg potassium, 2g fiber

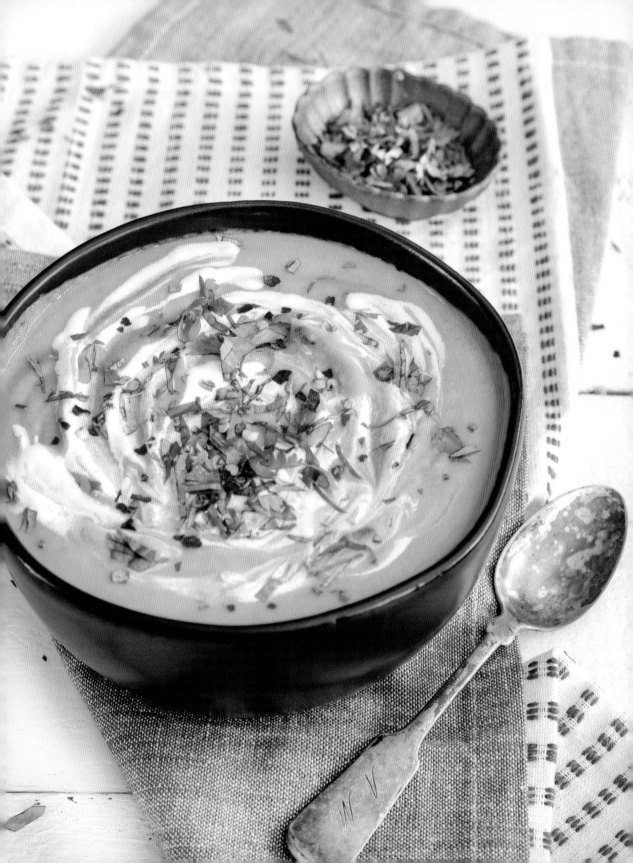

Weekend Meals

Before I was diagnosed with migraine disease, I cooked on the fly with no meal planning. I still don't do weekly meal planning, but I find that spending a couple of hours cooking on the weekend makes my week a little easier. Some of these recipes are in bulk, so they'll make a lot of food to freeze in smaller portions, perfect for packable lunches for the office. Feel free to make the quicker ones on a weeknight too!

Carrot-Ginger Soup

When a neighbor offered me some carrot-ginger soup, I found the combination of sweet carrots, fresh ginger, turmeric, and a little heat from the red pepper flakes to be dynamite. Not to mention the anti-inflammatory benefits of turmeric and ginger. It might be my favorite recipe in this book, the best kind of medicine in a bowl.

Makes 8 servings

Prep time: 30 minutes
Cooking time: 40 minutes
                (stovetop)
                15 minutes
                (Instant Pot)
Passive time: N/A

Budget friendly: Very

2 tablespoons extra-virgin olive oil

2 pounds (1kg) carrots, peeled and roughly chopped

2 large leeks, cleaned, roughly chopped (white and light-green parts only)

2 cloves garlic, peeled

2 tablespoons minced fresh ginger root

1 tablespoon ground turmeric

2 teaspoons ground cumin

¼ teaspoon red pepper flakes (see Cook's Note)

½ teaspoon white pepper

4 cups (.95L) low-sodium chicken or vegetable broth

1 (14.5-ounce [428mL]) can regular coconut milk

1 cup (50g) finely chopped cilantro or fresh Italian parsley

Stovetop instructions:

1 Heat the olive oil in a large heavy-bottom pot or Dutch oven over medium-high heat. Add the carrots and leeks; sauté until leeks begin to soften, about 5 minutes.

2 Add the garlic, ginger, turmeric, cumin, red pepper flakes, and pepper. Sauté for 1 to 2 minutes.

3 Add the broth. Bring to a boil and reduce heat, simmering uncovered until vegetables are fork-tender, about 30 minutes.

4 Remove from heat and stir in the coconut milk, until all solids have melted.

5 Puree the soup until perfectly smooth. See box on the next page.

6 Stir in the herbs and serve at once.

Instant Pot instructions:

1 Select Sauté (normal heat), add the oil, and sauté the carrots and leeks for 5 minutes, stirring often. Press Cancel.

2 Add the garlic, ginger, turmeric, cumin, red pepper flakes, and pepper; sauté for 1 to 2 minutes. Secure the lid.

3 Select Pressure Cook at high pressure for 8 minutes.

4 Use the quick release, covering the vent with a kitchen towel to avoid splatters.

5 Stir in the coconut milk, allowing the heat to melt any solids.

6 Follow Steps 5 and 6 above to finish the soup.

 If lemons are not a trigger for you, a squeeze of lemon juice adds a lovely tang.

PER 1-CUP SERVING: 2g protein, 12g carbohydrates, 8g fat, 6g saturated fat, 69mg sodium, 302mg potassium, 3g fiber

BLENDING HOT SOUP: *If using a regular blender, blend in batches, and cover the top with a kitchen towel to protect yourself from the escaping steam. If using an immersion blender, place a hot pad under the pot on the counter and with another, hold the pot at an angle away from you. Blend the soup until very smooth.*

COOK'S NOTE: *This soup freezes beautifully. If using frozen or pre-cleaned leeks, you'll need 2 cups sliced (180g). Reserve the green tops from the cleaned leeks to make Beany-Brothy Deliciousness (p. 142) or Low-Sodium Chicken Broth (p. 136). If you don't like spice, omit the red pepper flakes, or start with ⅛ teaspoon. Cilantro and fresh parsley bunches will vary in size. Feel free to use the entire bunch of either; it will not affect the taste.*

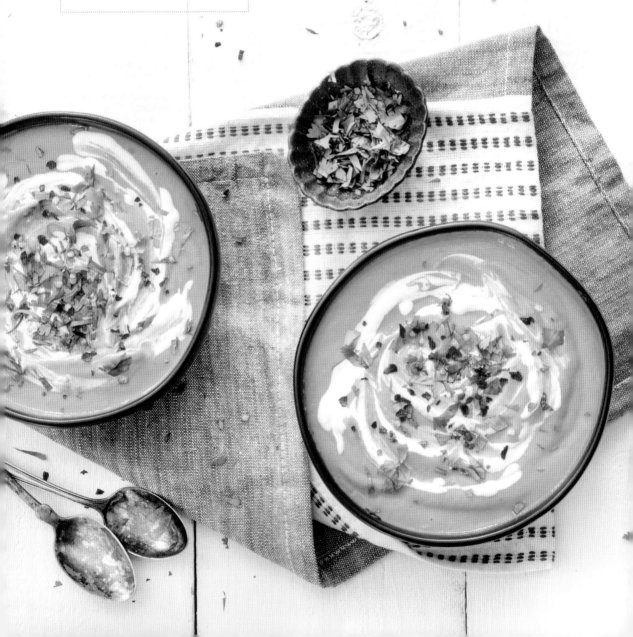

Creamy Potato Soup

Being of German heritage, my mom cooked potatoes multiple times a week. Ham and scalloped potatoes were her way of stretching leftovers further. There's no Velveeta cheese in here, but this soup has the same comforting, nostalgic taste as that dish. I use the reduced-sodium ham sparingly, for flavor, and a mild chile pepper adds a little kick.

Makes 4 servings

Prep time: 20 minutes
Cooking time: 30 minutes
Passive time: 30 minutes

Budget friendly: Very

1 pound (450g) red or russet potatoes, peeled and cut into evenly sized chunks

2 cloves garlic, crushed

6 ounces (175g) fresh Hatch or Anaheim mild chile peppers (See Cook's Note for using frozen or canned)

2 ounces (50g) reduced-sodium uncured ham (optional), diced

1 cup (250mL) Low-Sodium Chicken Broth (p. 136)

1 cup (250mL) canned coconut milk or organic half and half

½ teaspoon ground cumin

⅛ teaspoon white pepper

1 pinch cinnamon

1 Cover cut potatoes in cold water for at least 30 minutes to reduce starch content in the finished soup.

2 Meanwhile, prepare the chiles if using fresh: Broil until peppers are black, put in a paper bag until cool, then peel, seed, and de-stem. Roughly chop. Set aside a few chiles for garnish, if desired.

3 Drain the potatoes and add them to a saucepan with the garlic. Cover with filtered water and bring to a boil. Boil for 10 to 15 minutes until fork tender.

4 Sauté the ham (if using) in a nonstick pan until golden brown. Set aside a few pieces for garnishing the soup.

5 Drain the potatoes, add to a blender with the chicken broth, and puree just until smooth. Do not overwork or the soup becomes gummy.

6 Put the soup back in the saucepan with the coconut milk, ham (if using), chiles, and spices. Simmer for 15 minutes, until the soup is completely infused with flavor.

7 Ladle into bowls and top with the reserved ham and pepper garnishes. Serve at once.

COOK'S NOTE: *If using frozen chiles, thaw and drain ¾ cup prior to beginning this recipe. If using a 6-ounce can, do not drain.*

PER SERVING (with fresh chiles, ham, and coconut milk):
7g protein, 21g carbohydrates, 9g fat, 8g saturated fat, 180mg sodium, 664mg potassium, 2g fiber

PER SERVING (with fresh chiles and coconut milk):
5g protein, 21g carbohydrates, 9g fat, 8g saturated fat, 48mg sodium, 664mg potassium, 2g fiber

Detox Veggie Soup

While the jury is still out on whether it's possible to "detox" the body using food, veggie-packed soups are undeniably a recipe for feeling better after a period of indulgence. This soup isn't going to win a beauty contest. When I'm craving nutrition after overdoing it (holiday season, anyone?) this is just the thing.

Makes 8 servings

Prep time: 20 minutes
Cooking time: 40 minutes
Passive time: N/A

Budget friendly: Very

4 medium or 3 large zucchini

4 kale leaves, stems included

3 green onions

2 carrots

3 celery stalks

1 pound (450g) fresh green beans, trimmed

3 cloves garlic

2 cups (100g) fresh Italian parsley

1 cup (50g) packed cilantro

1 (14.5-ounce [411g]) can no-salt-added diced tomatoes

4 cups (.95L) water

1 Place all the produce and herbs except the tomatoes in the bowl of a food processor. Reserve a little chopped parsley for garnishing. Pulse until finely chopped.

2 Transfer to a large, heavy-bottomed pot and add the tomatoes and water.

3 Bring just to a boil, then reduce the heat, cover, and simmer gently for 30 minutes.

4 Serve and garnish with reserved parsley.

COOK'S NOTE: *Fresh basil can be substituted for cilantro. If you have access to home-grown or farmers' market tomatoes, use 3 tomatoes instead of the can and pulse them through the food processor.*

PER SERVING: 5g protein, 13g carbohydrates, 1g fat, 0g saturated fat, 69mg sodium, 574mg potassium, 5g fiber

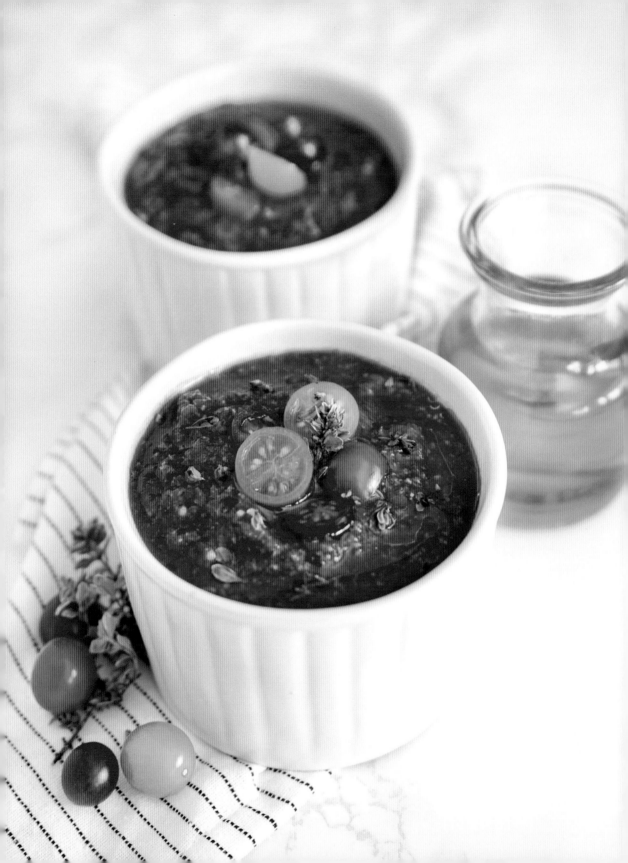

Gazpacho

For my 50th birthday, I took a trip to France. My first meal in Provence was a gazpacho served chilled in a mason jar and topped with salad. It remains one of my favorite food memories. Making this recipe brings back the flavors of that refreshing cold soup on a blistering hot day.

Serves 4

Prep time: 30 minutes
Cooking time: 5 minutes
Passive time: 30 minutes to
                        overnight

Budget friendly: Very

1 pound (450g) fresh garden or farmers' market tomatoes, roughly chopped

14 ounces (400g) cucumber, peeled, seeded, roughly chopped

8 ounces (225g) red bell peppers, stemmed and seeded, roughly chopped

2 tablespoons extra-virgin olive oil

2 teaspoons white vinegar

2 cloves garlic, minced or pressed

2 sprigs fresh savory, leaves only

2 sprigs fresh thyme, leaves only

1 slice gluten-free bread, well toasted

1 Mix all the ingredients except the bread in a large bowl. Refrigerate 30 minutes to overnight to let the flavors develop.

2 Process the cold vegetable mixture using a food processor or blender, leaving it a bit chunky.

3 Soak the bread in cold water for 20 minutes. Squeeze out the water and tear the bread into pieces.

4 Add the bread to the soup and pulse just until completely incorporated. Don't over-process or you'll lose the thickening the bread provides.

5 Serve cold.

COOK'S NOTE: *Use your best olive oil. If you use English or Persian cucumbers, skip the peeling and deseeding. Bright-red, store-bought organic cherry tomatoes are acceptable. Do not use regular grocery store tomatoes; the flavor will be supremely disappointing. Substitute ⅛ teaspoon each dried thyme and savory (or marjoram), or ¼ teaspoon no-salt-added Herbes de Provence for the fresh herbs.*

PER SERVING (with Trader Joe's Gluten-Free Multigrain Brown Rice Bread):
3g protein, 15g carbohydrates, 8g fat, 1g saturated fat, 27mg sodium, 429mg potassium, 1g fiber

Parsnip-Leek Soup

Parsnips look like knobby white carrots and are nearly as sweet with a lovely earthy taste. Pairing them with nutmeg, sage, and white pepper creates a soup that's creamy and light, spicy and delicious. Varying the vegetables I eat helps make sure I'm getting a range of nutrients from my meals.

Makes 6 servings

Prep time:	20 minutes
Cooking time:	45 minutes to 1 hour on stovetop; 15 to 20 minutes in Instant Pot (including time it takes to come to pressure)
Passive time:	N/A

Budget friendly: Very

1 tablespoon extra-virgin olive oil

4 leeks, white parts only, cleaned and sliced

6 green onions, white parts only, thinly sliced

3 cloves garlic, minced

4 parsnips (450-500g), peeled and roughly chopped

½ teaspoon ground nutmeg

½ teaspoon dried sage

¼ teaspoon white pepper

4 cups (.95L) Low-Sodium Vegetable Broth (p. 204) or Low-Sodium Chicken Broth (p. 136)

Stovetop instructions:

1 Heat the olive oil in a large heavy-bottomed soup pot over medium-high heat. Stir in the leeks and green onions. Cook for 8 minutes or until leeks have wilted. Add the garlic and cook 1 minute longer.

2 Add the parsnips, nutmeg, sage, and white pepper. Cook for 3 more minutes, stirring as needed to prevent sticking.

3 Add the broth. Cover and bring just to a boil, then reduce the heat to a gentle simmer and cook for 30 to 45 minutes, until the parsnips are very tender.

4 Puree until completely smooth. (See box on page 75 for safety tips when blending hot soups.)

Instant Pot instructions:

1 Select Sauté (normal heat) and cook the leeks and green onions in the oil for 5 minutes. Press Cancel.

2 Add the garlic and sauté 1 minute.

3 Stir in the remaining ingredients. Secure the lid. Select Pressure Cook at high pressure for 5 minutes.

4 Use a quick release, covering the vent with a kitchen towel to avoid hot splatters.

5 Puree until completely smooth. (See box on page 75 for safety tips when blending hot soups.)

 If lemons are not a trigger for you, a squeeze of lemon adds the perfect amount of acidity.

PER SERVING (with low-sodium vegetable broth):
3g protein, 25g carbohydrates, 5g fat, 1g saturated fat, 101mg sodium, 421mg potassium, 6g fiber

"The moments in my life that I have had the most difficulty have also been the moments that I have found the wildest, inspired creation. And those are the moments when I've become more myself. I dive deeper into who I am and what I want and who I will become. Those are the moments that we find our purpose, where we confront our maker."

ALEXIS DONKIN, WRITER AND LONG-COVID PATIENT

COOK'S NOTE: *To clean leeks: Slice lengthwise, stopping before the root. Hold upside down under running water and pull open the leek's layers, washing out the dirt. Shake dry. Reserve the green parts of the leeks and green onions in a zip-top bag in the freezer for making Low-Sodium Chicken Broth (p. 136) or Beany-Brothy Deliciousness (p. 142). If using frozen or pre-cleaned leeks, use 6 cups sliced (400g).*

Spicy Sweet Potato Soup

I used to make slow-cooker chicken with a jar of salsa verde and throw sweet potatoes on top. Blending the leftover cooked sweet potatoes with the liquid from the pot made an outstanding soup, so I created this recipe to replicate that flavor.

Makes 6 servings

Prep time: 15 minutes
Cooking time: 30 minutes
Passive time: N/A

Budget friendly: Very

2 tablespoons extra-virgin olive oil

13 ounces (375g) sweet potatoes (about 3 cups), peeled and roughly chopped

2 cloves garlic, roughly chopped or pressed

1 teaspoon smoked paprika

4 cups (.95L) no-salt-added vegetable or chicken broth

1 (4-ounce [113g]) can diced fire-roasted mild green chiles

Stovetop instructions:

1 In a large sauce pan or Dutch oven with a lid, warm the oil over medium heat. Add the sweet potatoes and sauté for 9 minutes. Add the garlic and smoked paprika and cook for 1 to 2 minutes, until garlic is lightly browned.

2 Add the broth and chiles, cover and bring just to a boil, then reduce heat to a simmer. Cook a few minutes more, checking every 5 minutes, until the sweet potatoes are fork tender.

3 Blend the soup until smooth (see box on page 75). Garnish as desired (see Cook's Note) and serve at once.

Instant Pot instructions:

1 Select Sauté (normal heat), add the oil, and cook the sweet potatoes for 5 minutes, stirring frequently. Press Cancel.

2 Add the garlic and smoked paprika and sauté 1 minute.

3 Stir in the remaining ingredients and secure the lid.

4 Select Pressure Cook at high pressure for 5 minutes.

5 Use a quick release, covering the valve with a kitchen towel to avoid hot splatters.

6 Follow Step 3 above to complete the recipe.

COOK'S NOTE: *Garnish with minced cilantro or Italian parsley, toasted pumpkin seeds, chèvre, or gluten-free croutons. This soup freezes well. A 3- or 4-quart pot is the best size for this recipe. If you don't like heat, omit the green chiles or substitute a roasted bell pepper. If canned, diced green chiles are not available, use 1 or 2 medium-heat fresh green chile peppers. The recipe will work for 12 to 16 ounces (340–450g) of sweet potato. One tester suggested adding minced shallot during Step 1 for even richer flavor.*

PER SERVING (with low-sodium vegetable broth):
1g protein, 12g carbohydrates, 4g fat, 1g saturated fat, 86mg sodium, 194mg potassium, 1g fiber

"Resilience is finding a way back to yourself. As we go through more experiences in life, there are more traumas. We eventually have the arsenal of tools that we're able to use to spring back into who we were, or at least where we were before the event. There was no way I was ever going to go back to the life I had before getting hit by that truck, but who I was as Marisa at my core, that's what I had to figure out how to get back to. If everything is taken away from you, who are you with nothing?"

**MARISA ZEPPIERI, AUTHOR OF *CHRONICALLY FABULOUS:
FINDING WHOLENESS AND HOPE LIVING WITH CHRONIC ILLNESS***

Twice-Baked Thai-Spiced Potatoes

I loved the Samosa Stuffed Baked Potatoes in *Veganomicon* by Isa Chandra Moskowitz and Terry Hope Romero, who added an array of spices and ingredients to mirror the flavor of a samosa. I thought, why not a version using Thai curry paste? This rich recipe is filling enough for dinner on its own. I use leftovers, if there are any, to make potato patties by mashing them in a bowl with an egg or two and lightly frying in a sauté pan until crisp.

Makes 4 servings

Prep time: 30 minutes
Cooking time: 2 hours
Passive time: 1 hour

Budget-friendly: Very

2 large or 4 small baking potatoes, scrubbed (See Cook's Note)

1 tablespoon coconut oil

2 tablespoons Thai (Green or Red) Curry Paste (p. 198), or store-bought

1 cup (250mL) canned coconut milk, divided

½ cup (70g) fresh or frozen peas

1 large carrot, or 10 baby carrots, diced

¼ red bell pepper, diced

PER SERVING (with commercial Thai green curry paste; sodium will be far lower if you make your own): 5g protein, 40g carbohydrates, 6g fat, 2g saturated fat, 223mg sodium, 902mg potassium, 4g fiber

1 Preheat oven to 400°F (200°C).

2 Prick the potatoes with a fork, then wrap in foil and bake for 60 to 80 minutes, until soft. Leave the oven on. Cool the potatoes long enough to handle them without burning yourself.

3 While the potatoes are cooling, heat the coconut oil in a deep saucepan over medium heat until shimmering. Add the Thai green curry paste and fry for 2 minutes until very fragrant. Protect yourself with a lid or splatter guard when adding the curry paste.

4 Stir ½ cup of the coconut milk into the curry paste until thoroughly blended.

5 Add the peas and carrots and cook for 5 minutes until almost boiling. Add the peppers and cook another 5 minutes, until carrots are still firm but not crunchy.

6 When the potatoes are cool enough to handle, cut them in half lengthwise along the narrower side to create boats. With a grapefruit spoon or paring knife, remove the centers of the cooked potatoes, leaving about ¼ inch (6 to 8 mm) around the edge. Take your time; it's easy to break the edge or poke through the bottom.

7 Mash the potato centers in a large bowl with a fork or potato masher. Add the remaining ½ cup of the coconut milk a little at a time, until very smooth but still a little dry. Season with a tiny bit of salt and black pepper to taste.

8 Mix in the curry veggies, combining well without smushing the peas.

9 With an ice cream scoop, round measuring cup, or large spoon, pack the mixture evenly into the four potato skins. Spray lightly with olive or coconut oil spray. Bake in a heatproof dish for 15 minutes, or until heated through and golden brown on top.

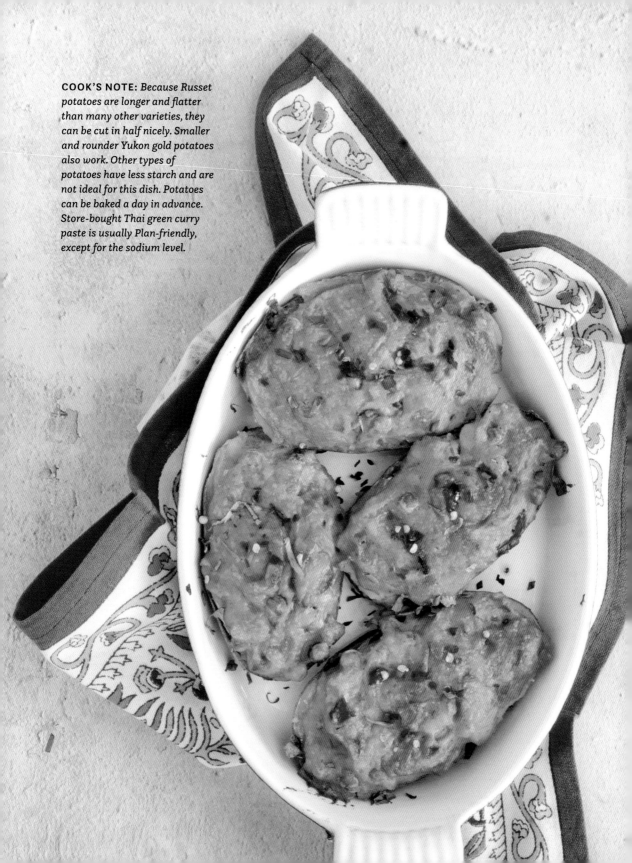

COOK'S NOTE: *Because Russet potatoes are longer and flatter than many other varieties, they can be cut in half nicely. Smaller and rounder Yukon gold potatoes also work. Other types of potatoes have less starch and are not ideal for this dish. Potatoes can be baked a day in advance. Store-bought Thai green curry paste is usually Plan-friendly, except for the sodium level.*

South Asian-Inspired Chickpea Masala

This is a hearty vegetarian curry rich in flavor but not overly spicy. In Pakistan, Nepal, India, and Bangladesh, *masala* refers to a mixture of ground spices.

Makes 4–5 servings

Prep time:	30 minutes
Cooking time:	45 minutes
Passive time:	N/A

Budget friendly: Very

2 tablespoons extra-virgin olive oil

1 leek, washed and thinly sliced (or 1 cup [90g] frozen prepared leeks)

2 large carrots, diced

4 cloves garlic, minced

3 bay leaves

2 teaspoons garam masala, either a no-salt-added store-bought version or mine (p. 199)

1 teaspoon ground cumin

½ teaspoon chipotle powder

1 (13.5-ounce [400mL]) can light coconut milk

1 (6-ounce [170g]) can no-salt-added tomato paste

1 (15-ounce [425g]) can low-sodium or no-salt-added chickpeas, drained

¾ cup (50g) kale, chopped

1 Heat the oil in a large sauté pan over medium heat until shimmering. Cook the leek, carrots, garlic, bay leaves, and spices for 10 minutes.

2 Add the remaining ingredients plus 13.5 ounces (400mL) filtered water (use the coconut-milk can) and stir well.

3 Bring almost to a boil, then reduce the heat to a gentle bubble. Cook uncovered for 20 to 30 minutes.

4 Remove the 3 bay leaves before serving.

COOK'S NOTE: *Some recipe testers reduced the tomato paste and coconut milk to their liking. One tester who is diabetic uses chana dal, a type of split chickpea that has the lowest score on the glycemic index (8). For a diabetic-friendly version of this dish, cook your own chana dal first in an Instant Pot. Add 1 cup chana dal (rinsed well) and 4 cups (.95L) filtered water; secure the lid. Pressure Cook on high pressure for 6 minutes. Press Cancel, then use natural pressure release. Total cook time is about one hour.*

SERVING SUGGESTIONS: Serve over brown rice, Saffron Rice (p. 120), or with Coconut-Curried Greens (p. 110).

PER 1-CUP SERVING: 6g protein, 23g carbohydrates, 16g fat, 8g saturated fat, 58mg sodium, 411mg potassium, 5g fiber

Spicy Black Bean and Rice Casserole

When the weather is cool, I am all about the one-dish casseroles. Maybe it's because I grew up Lutheran, and potluck dinners were a regular event. This hearty recipe is so packed with veggies, protein, and smoky spices, you won't miss the meat. Adjust the spice level to suit your taste.

Makes 6–8 side dish servings

Prep time: 10 minutes
Cooking time: 50–55 minutes
Passive time: 10 minutes

Budget friendly: Very

Cooking spray or oil for greasing baking dish

6 ounces (175g) fresh spinach

4 green onions

8 ounces (250g) whole milk or part-skim ricotta cheese

4 eggs

2 teaspoons smoked paprika

2 teaspoons ground cumin

2 teaspoons garlic powder or granulated garlic

½ teaspoon freshly ground black pepper

¼ teaspoon chipotle powder, or to taste (optional)

¼ teaspoon liquid smoke (optional)

2 cups (400g) cooked brown rice

1 (15.5-ounce [450g]) can no-salt-added black beans, rinsed and drained well

1 Preheat the oven to 350°F (180°C).

2 Spray or oil an oven-proof 9 × 11-inch (23 × 33cm) baking dish or a deep 9-inch (23cm) pie pan.

3 Pulse the spinach and green onions in a food processor until roughly chopped.

4 In a large mixing bowl, stir in the ricotta, eggs, spices, and liquid smoke (if using) until well blended. Stir in the chopped spinach mixture, brown rice, and beans, and continue mixing until evenly coated.

5 Spoon into the prepared pan and smooth the top.

6 Bake for 50 to 55 minutes until top is golden brown, firm, and bounces back when lightly pressed in the center. The center should not jiggle.

7 Cool on a wire rack for 10 minutes before serving.

COOK'S NOTE: *Black-eyed peas can be substituted for the black beans. If you can't find canned beans without salt, cook your own using the method on page 142. Up to a cup of diced or shredded chicken can be added in Step 4.*

SERVING SUGGESTIONS: Add something green to your plate, such as Coconut-Curried Greens (p. 110), Pan-Roasted Kale with Crispy Italian Breadcrumbs (p. 129), or Spicy Kale and Swiss Chard Sauté (p. 243, *The Migraine Relief Plan*).

PER SERVING: 10g protein, 19g carbohydrates, 6g fat, 3g saturated fat, 58mg sodium, 307 mg potassium, 3g fiber

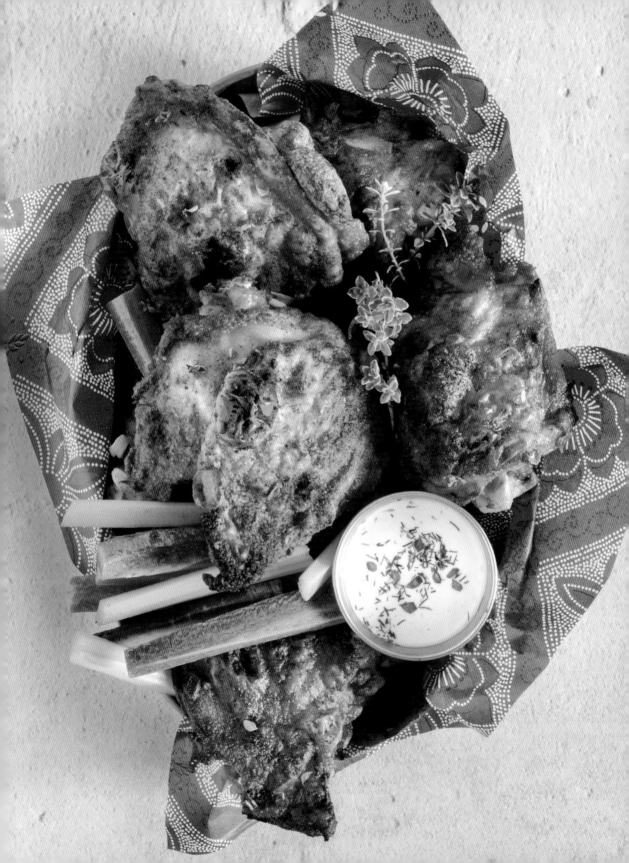

Sheet Pan Chicken Thighs

Once this goes in the oven it's almost completely hands-off. The skin turns out exquisitely crispy and the meat is incredibly juicy. Use a rimmed half-sheet pan, not a cookie sheet, for this recipe. A favorite of even the pickiest kids!

Makes 8 servings

Prep time:	10 minutes
Cooking time:	30 minutes
Passive time:	N/A

Budget friendly: Very

¼ cup (32g) coconut flour

2 teaspoons smoked paprika

2 teaspoons garlic powder

½ teaspoon white pepper

¼ teaspoon chipotle or cayenne powder

¼ teaspoon smoked salt (optional)

8 bone-in, skin-on chicken thighs

Olive or coconut oil spray (see Cook's Note)

1 Preheat the oven to 400°F (200°C).

2 Mix the dry ingredients in a large zip-top bag or bowl with a tight-fitting lid. Add the chicken and shake until lightly and evenly coated. If chicken thighs are large, coat in 2 batches. Throw out leftover coating mixture.

3 Place chicken on a sheet pan covered in aluminum foil and spray or drizzle chicken lightly with oil.

4 Place pan in the oven and roast for 25 minutes. Remove pan from oven and carefully mop up excess oil with a paper towel and tongs before flipping thighs over.

5 Rotate pan and bake another 20 minutes. Chicken should register at least 165°F (74°C) in the thickest part of the thigh.

COOK'S NOTE: *If you don't have cooking spray, lightly drizzle the oil over the chicken. Lining the pan with foil makes clean-up a breeze. Bone-in, skin-on thighs are inexpensive cuts and provide rich flavor. Thighs will vary in weight from 5 to 8 ounces, which will affect your cooking time. Penzeys' Roasted Garlic Powder can be used instead of regular garlic powder.*

SERVING SUGGESTIONS: Choose two of my Scrumptious Sides (p. 109) and add a big green salad.

PER SERVING (with smoked salt):
22g protein, 2g carbohydrates, 19g fat, 6g saturated fat, 180mg sodium, 259mg potassium, 1g fiber.
106mg sodium if made without salt.

Lazy Chicken and Broth

I make this very simple meal once a week for my husband. As a bonus, this cooking method leaves you with collagen-rich, low-sodium broth to use later.

Makes 16 servings of meat and approximately 2 cups of broth

Prep time: 5 minutes
Cooking time: 4–5 hours in
                 the slow cooker;
                 about an hour in
                 the Instant Pot
Passive time: N/A

Budget friendly: Moderate

4 pounds (1.8kg) bone-in chicken (see Cook's Note)

2 tablespoons mild or medium chili powder

Slow-cooker instructions (6 quart):

1 Sprinkle the chicken pieces with the chili powder on all sides.

2 Set to low. Put breast pieces (if using) skin-side-down in the bottom, drumsticks on top. Cover and cook for 4 to 5 hours, or until meat falls off the bone.

3 Remove the chicken with tongs, then pour the broth into a container to use for soup or other recipes.

Instant Pot instructions (6 quart):

1 Sprinkle the chicken pieces with the chili powder on all sides.

2 Place 1 cup (240mL) filtered water in bottom and add rack. Place the chicken pieces directly on the rack. Secure the lid. Select Pressure Cook at high pressure for 22 minutes, then wait 15 minutes before releasing the pressure. Follow Step 3 above to complete the recipe.

COOK'S NOTE: *I use one family-size split breast pack of chicken, which includes 2 split breasts and 4 drumsticks, then add 2 more packages of drumsticks. If you prefer dark meat, use 3 packages of drumsticks, which are the least expensive cut, even for organic chicken. I tested a whole chicken and it came out perfectly.*

SERVING SUGGESTIONS: Dice chicken breast and use for Curried Chicken Salad (p. 56) or Mango Chicken Salad (p. 54). Top Fattoush Salad (p. 59) with shredded meat or enjoy it as is with any two Scrumptious Sides (p. 109).

PER 4-OUNCE SERVING (one organic drumstick):
20g protein, 0g carbohydrates, 10g fat, 3g saturated fat, 95mg sodium, 0mg potassium, 0g fiber

Cozy Chicken and Rice

One of my readers shared a version of this favorite that she'd originally clipped from the *New York Times*. I've perfected it for the Plan. Put in less than 10 minutes of prep time, then set a timer and enjoy a satisfying dinner 40 minutes later.

Makes 6 servings

Prep time: 10 minutes
Cooking time: 40 minutes
Passive time: N/A

Budget friendly: Very

2 tablespoons butter or extra-virgin olive oil

10 ounces (285g) white or cremini mushrooms, sliced

1 (6-ounce [170g]) bunch green onions (about 16), thinly sliced

3 bay leaves

1 ¼ pounds (550g) boneless, skinless chicken thighs, snipped into chunks

2 cloves garlic, smashed and chopped

2 tablespoons white wine (optional)

1 cup (240g) basmati rice, rinsed 3 times and drained thoroughly

2 cups (480mL) Low-Sodium Chicken Broth (p. 136), heated until nearly boiling

6 ounces (170g) baby spinach

1 Heat the butter or olive oil in a large nonstick sauté pan with a lid over medium heat.

2 Sauté the mushrooms, green onions, and bay leaves (uncovered) until mushrooms are golden and have released their liquid, about 10 minutes. Mushrooms should be dry and golden brown.

3 Add the chicken, garlic, and wine (if using). Sauté for 5 minutes until wine is gone.

4 Push vegetables and chicken to the edges of the pan and add the rice in the center.

5 Gently pour in the heated broth, making sure rice is immersed. Adjust heat so that rice is just bubbling. Cover pan and cook for 20 minutes or until the rice is tender. Remove bay leaves.

6 Sprinkle spinach on top, cover, and cook 3 minutes until wilted. Stir well.

7 Turn off heat. Serve while still warm.

COOK'S NOTE: *You can substitute 2 diced shallots for the green onions, and well-rinsed white or jasmine rice for the basmati. The longer cooking time required for brown rice does not provide consistent results in this recipe.*

SERVING SUGGESTIONS: I tend to eat one-dish meals like this on their own, but adding a big green salad balances out the richness of the chicken thighs.

PER 1¼-CUP SERVING (with unsalted butter):
24g protein, 28g carbohydrates, 9g fat, 3g saturated fat, 114mg sodium, 386mg potassium, 3g fiber

White Chicken Chili

I first tasted white chili, (so named because of the absence of tomatoes), at a chili cook-off that's become a neighborhood tradition. Here's my Plan-friendly version featuring white kidney (cannellini) beans, green onions, and green chile peppers.

Makes 6 servings

Prep time: 5 minutes
Cooking time: 35 minutes
Passive time: N/A

Budget friendly: Very

2 tablespoons extra-virgin olive oil

1 (6-ounce [170g]) bunch green onions (about 16), whites only, chopped

2 cloves garlic, minced

1 teaspoon chili powder

1 teaspoon ground cumin

1 teaspoon dried oregano

½ teaspoon freshly ground black pepper

4 cups (320g) diced or shredded cooked chicken breast

2 (15.5-ounce [439g]) cans no-salt-added white cannellini beans, 1 can pureed with its juice, the other rinsed and drained

1 (4-ounce [113g]) can fire-roasted diced green chile peppers, not drained

1 cup (240mL) no-salt-added chicken or vegetable broth

Minced cilantro, for garnishing

Stovetop instructions:

1 In a large skillet with a lid, heat the oil over medium heat and sauté the green onions for 5 minutes. Add the garlic and spices and stir one minute more.

2 Add the remaining ingredients and stir well.

3 Bring just to a boil over medium-high heat, then reduce heat to low, cover, and simmer 30 minutes, stirring every 10 minutes. Add additional broth if it gets too thick or begins to stick.

4 Divide into bowls and garnish with cilantro, if desired.

Slow-cooker instructions:

1 Combine all the ingredients and cook on low for at least 4 hours.

Instant Pot instructions:

1 Sauté the green onions and garlic on Sauté setting (low) for 5 minutes. Press Cancel. Stir in the rest of the ingredients and press Slow Cooker. Close but do not pressurize lid. Cook for 4 hours.

COOK'S NOTE: *If you only find 7-ounce cans of green chiles, use the whole can. Canned beans can range from 14.5 to 15.5 ounces; use what you find. If you like spice, amp up the flavor with additional chili powder, cumin, and black or white pepper. Try cooking beans using Beany-Brothy Deliciousness (p. 142). Use leftover chicken from Lazy Chicken (p. 90) or Roasted Chicken with Veggie Gravy (p. 134).*

PER 1-CUP SERVING:
25g protein, 25g carbohydrates, 6g fat, 1g saturated fat, 170mg sodium, 735mg potassium, 8g fiber

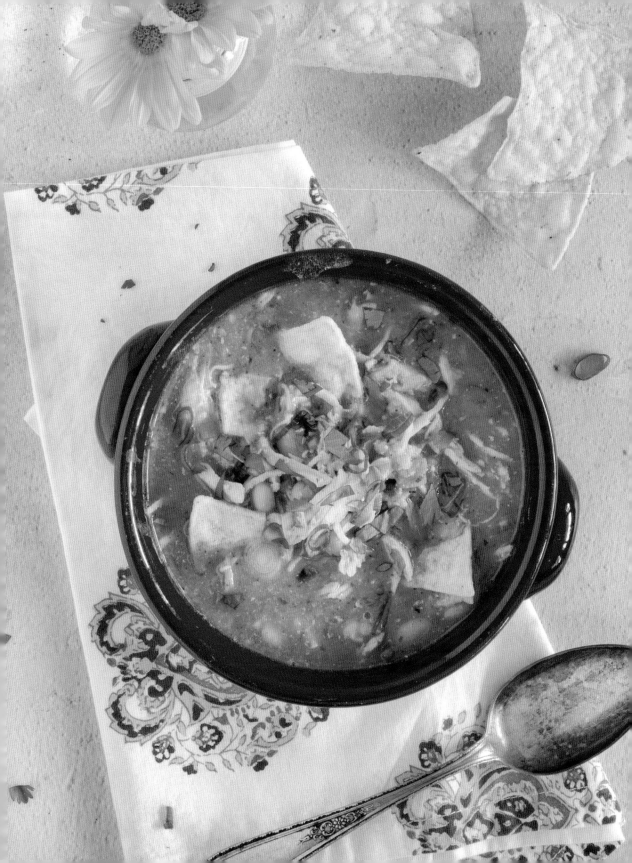

Turkey Mole Tamale Pie

I have always adored tamales, but making them is an all-day affair and requires more skill with corn husks than I have. While it's the most time-intensive dish in the book, if you love the texture of tamales and the flavor of a chocolate-style Mexican mole, you'll find this pie worth the effort. Note that this is not an authentic Mexican dish; it's inspired by Mexican flavor profiles. It can be made vegan or vegetarian if you prefer.

Makes 6–8 servings

Prep time: 30 minutes
Cooking time: 90 minutes
Passive time: N/A

Budget friendly: Very
(if you have the spices)

2 ½ tablespoons chili powder

1 tablespoon unsweetened carob powder

2 teaspoons ground cumin

1 teaspoon ground cinnamon

1 teaspoon dried oregano

¼ teaspoon ground cloves

¼ teaspoon cayenne, ground red pepper, or chipotle powder

2 tablespoons extra-virgin olive or coconut oil, divided

12 green onions, thinly sliced

1¼ pounds (565g) ground turkey

3 cloves garlic, minced, divided

1½ cups (185g) butternut squash or sweet potato, peeled and cubed

1 red bell pepper, chopped

2 stalks celery, chopped

1 (14.5-ounce [411g]) can of no-salt-added diced tomatoes or tomato puree

3½ cups (840mL) filtered water

1⅓ cups (210g) stoneground yellow cornmeal

¼ teaspoon freshly ground black pepper

2 tablespoons chopped cilantro (optional)

4 ounces (113g) chèvre, crumbled (optional)

PER SERVING: 17g protein, 26g carbohydrates, 10g fat, 2g saturated fat, 113mg sodium, 493mg potassium, 5g fiber

1 Mix the 7 spices in a bowl until completely incorporated.

2 Add the oil to two deep nonstick or cast-iron frying pans on medium-high heat.

3 Cook half the green onions in each pan for 5 minutes, stirring occasionally, until golden.

4 Pan #1: Add the meat, half the garlic, and half the spice mixture, stirring to mix thoroughly. Cook until browned and broken up, about 10 minutes. Turn off the heat.

5 Pan #2: Add the squash, red pepper, celery, tomatoes, the rest of the garlic, and the remaining spice mixture, stirring thoroughly to combine. Cover the pan and cook until squash is just fork tender, 15 to 20 minutes.

6 Preheat the oven to 350°F (180°C).

7 Bring the water to a boil in a saucepan and whisk in the cornmeal. Turn the burner down to medium. Cook for 7 to 10 minutes, whisking frequently until very thick.

8 Mix the contents of each pan together in an oven-safe 12-inch frying pan or an oiled ovenproof casserole dish.

9 Stir the black pepper and optional cilantro and/or chèvre into the cornmeal mixture. Use a spatula to spread it evenly over the top of the meat and vegetable mixture.

10 Bake for 45 minutes or until top is browned. Let sit 5 to 10 minutes before serving.

COOK'S NOTE: *Masa can be substituted for cornmeal; it is sold in the Latin foods section of most large grocery stores. For quicker assembly, prep ingredients the day before. Substitute ground pork or chicken for the turkey. Omit ingredients in frying Pan #1 and increase the veggies to make this vegan.*

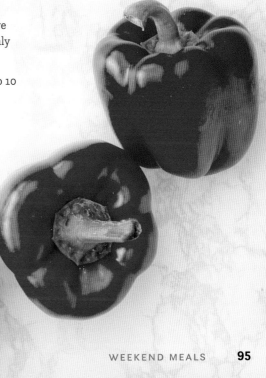

Slow-Cooker Turkey Breast

Store-bought turkey breast tends to be high in sodium. I wanted to create an easy way to make your own turkey breast for sandwiches or other recipes, like my Quick Turkey Tacos (page 98). I experimented with several ideas until coming up with this method, which takes just 10 minutes of prep and then goes in the slow cooker, coming out perfectly juicy and beautifully seasoned.

Makes 8 servings

Prep time: 10 minutes
Cooking time: 4 hours
Passive time: N/A

Budget friendly: Moderate

2 pounds (907g) bone-in turkey breast, cut into 2–3 pieces

1 tablespoon extra-virgin olive oil

1 teaspoon garlic powder

1 teaspoon dried cumin

1 teaspoon smoked paprika

½ teaspoon freshly ground black pepper

¼ teaspoon dried sage

1 Rub the turkey breast pieces on all sides with the olive oil.

2 Mix the spices together in a small bowl, then season the turkey breast evenly.

3 Wrap each piece of turkey tightly in its own piece of foil, then place in a slow cooker on low for 4 hours.

COOK'S NOTE: *You do not need to place any water inside the slow cooker. You can include turkey legs or wings as well if they will fit. Ask the butcher to cut pieces for you if needed (they will do this at no charge). If you can only find deboned turkey breast, check for doneness after 3 hours, as it will cook more quickly. To make turkey sandwiches from the turkey breast, let it cool, remove and discard skin, then thinly slice.*

PER 4-OUNCE SERVING: 27g protein, 1g carbohydrates, 3g fat, 0g saturated fat, 16mg sodium, 319mg potassium, 0g fiber

"Literature has always played a significant role in my journey toward self-care. I can leave everything else behind and become completely absorbed. Another avenue is walking and spending time with my two golden retrievers, who are certified therapy dogs. They help ground me and provide a service to others, both of which contribute to my wellbeing."

KATHY O'SHEA, AUTHOR OF *MUCH MORE THAN A HEADACHE: UNDERSTANDING MIGRAINE THROUGH LITERATURE*

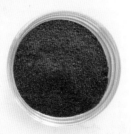 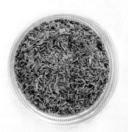 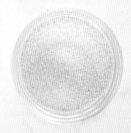

Quick Turkey Tacos

An unexpected way to use up leftover holiday turkey. Setting up a taco bar means that individual family members can heap on their own non-Plan toppings, like cheddar cheese or sour cream. Leftovers are excellent over rice the next day.

Makes 4 tacos

Prep time:	10 minutes
Cooking time:	15 minutes
Passive time:	N/A

Budget friendly: Very

1 (14.5-ounce [411g]) can no-salt-added pinto beans, rinsed

¼ cup (60mL) chile pepper sauce (see Cook's Note)

2–4 tablespoons filtered water

2 tablespoons extra-virgin coconut or olive oil

1 red bell pepper, thinly sliced

6 green onions, sliced diagonally

1 head baby bok choy, thinly sliced

1 clove garlic, minced

8 ounces (230g) cooked, shredded turkey breast

4 corn tortillas

1 Pulse the pinto beans in a food processor with the chile pepper sauce and 2 tablespoons of the filtered water until blended and the consistency of refried beans. Add water 1 tablespoon at a time if needed.

2 Place the bean mixture in a saucepan over low heat.

3 Heat the oil in a nonstick or cast-iron frying pan on medium-high heat until shimmering.

4 Sauté the vegetables and garlic until golden brown. Add the turkey and continue stirring until the meat is hot.

5 Toast the tortillas on a dry skillet or grill pan until lightly browned.

6 Fill the tortillas with the beans and the meat-vegetable mixture. Top with Hot Sauce (p. 196) if desired.

COOK'S NOTE: *If you do not have Chile Pepper Sauce (p. 267, The Migraine Relief Plan), whisk Hot Sauce (p. 196) into mayonnaise. If you don't have turkey left over from a holiday meal, make Slow-Cooker Turkey Breast (p. 96). I don't recommend grocery store rotisserie turkey as it's loaded with sodium. If doubling the recipe, do not double the bean/Chile Pepper Sauce ingredients. Feel free to substitute shredded chicken breast from Lazy Chicken (p. 90) or Roast Chicken with Veggie Gravy (p. 134) for the turkey. Note that the addition of baby bok choy, which proliferates in Asian cuisine, makes these non-traditional tacos.*

PER TACO (with low-sodium commercial turkey breast and Trader Joe's Chile Pepper Sauce):
19g protein, 34g carbohydrates, 8g fat, 0g saturated fat, 369mg sodium, 293mg potassium, 9g fiber

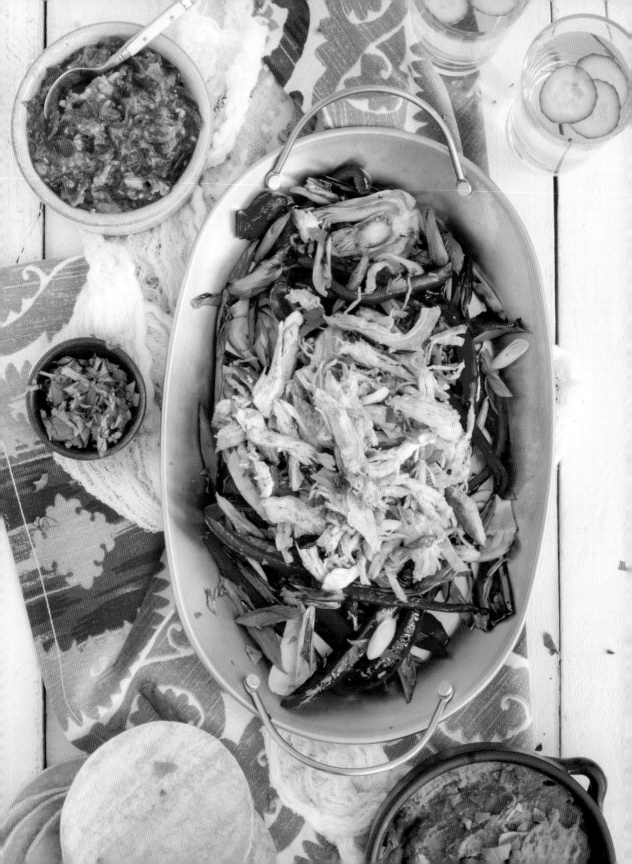

Super-Simple Beef Stew

When you're in pain, making food is a challenge. I wanted to speed up the prep on a beef stew without losing the flavor. I wash the potatoes right in the mesh bag, then put them straight into the slow cooker, along with the bag of baby carrots. Imagine coming home to a rich pot of beef stew.

Makes 6 servings

Prep time:	5 minutes
Cooking time:	8 hours
Passive time:	N/A

Budget friendly: Very

1 pound (500g) fingerling or
very small new potatoes

1 pound (500g) baby carrots

6 green onions, thinly sliced

1 (28-ounce [800g]) can no-
salt-added crushed or diced
tomatoes

1 pound (500g) grass-fed beef
pot roast, cubed

2 teaspoons ground cumin

2 teaspoons garlic powder

1 teaspoon freshly ground
black pepper

Slow-cooker instructions:

1 Add all the ingredients to a 6-quart slow cooker. Stir until thoroughly mixed.

2 Cover and cook on low for 7 to 8 hours.

Instant Pot instructions:

1 Combine all the ingredients in the pot. Stir well and cover.

2 Select Pressure Cook at high pressure for 25 minutes.

3 Use a natural pressure release for 20 minutes, then cover the valve with a kitchen towel before releasing remaining pressure.

COOK'S NOTE: *Ask the butcher to cut the meat for you into 1-inch chunks. The potatoes, green onions, and spices can be prepped the night before to save time. If you prefer a thicker stew, use 1 (14-ounce [400g]) can of tomatoes. This stew freezes well.*

SERVING SUGGESTIONS: If you run low-sodium cottage cheese through the blender, it tastes like sour cream and is lovely dolloped atop this stew. Serve with a green side salad and toasted gluten-free bread for dipping.

PER SERVING: 19g protein, 41g carbohydrates, 14g fat, 5g saturated fat, 77mg sodium, 330mg potassium, 7g fiber

"I write things down in my gratitude journal and tell people that I'm grateful for them on a regular basis. I pray every day for other people who I know are struggling with different things. Painting is a very meditative activity for me. When I'm painting, I have to focus carefully on my brush strokes and on mixing color. It clears my mind and takes me out of the worries of the day."

PAULA DUMAS, FOUNDER OF MIGRAINE AGAIN AND CO-HOST, MIGRAINE WORLD SUMMIT

Beef Barbacoa

If you love beef, this dish is worth the long simmering time. True Mexican barbacoa is made from marinated cuts of beef, lamb, or goat that have been steamed over hot coals in an underground pit. For this adapted recipe I use chuck roast, which is well-suited to my slow-cooker method. I also give instructions for Instant Pot and stovetop cooking. Whatever method you choose, don't skip the pan searing. I refrigerate enough for 2 or 3 days and freeze the remaining meat in labeled containers.

Makes 24 servings

Prep time:	5 minutes
Cooking time:	25 minutes for searing; 4–8 hours for braising
Passive time:	N/A

2 tablespoons mild chili powder

1 tablespoon smoked paprika

1 tablespoon granulated garlic

1 tablespoon dried oregano

¼–½ teaspoon chipotle powder, according to taste

2 tablespoons coconut oil

6 pounds (2.72kg) grass-fed beef chuck roast, cut into pieces approximately 2-inch × 3-inch × 4-inch (string removed if roast is tied)

1 (28-ounce [450g]) can no-salt-added crushed or pureed tomatoes

3 bay leaves

2 cups water or low-sodium broth (for Dutch oven method only)

Slow-cooker instructions:

1 Create a dry rub by mixing the first five ingredients together in a large shallow bowl until one color.

2 Dip the meat into the dry rub, massaging it in with your fingertips and shaking off excess until each piece is generously coated.

3 Heat the coconut oil in a large Dutch oven over medium heat until shimmering.

4 Place the meat into the Dutch oven and press down gently so that a flat surface forms. Do this in small batches, leaving about 2 inches between pieces, which allows them to brown and not steam. Cook until a brown crust has formed on the meat, approximately 1 to 2 minutes on each side. If the oil begins to smoke or spices begin to burn, reduce the heat. Set aside the Dutch oven for later.

5 Once each piece is seared, add it to an 8-quart slow cooker at a low setting.

6 Pour the tomatoes and any remaining spice mixture over the meat, add the bay leaves, and cover.

7 Cook for 4 to 6 hours until meat is tender and falls apart. Discard the bay leaves.

8 Place the beef in a large bowl and shred with two forks, removing any fatty portions or gristle. Pour the sauce back into the reserved Dutch oven or a saucepan and reduce, uncovered, over medium heat until thickened, about 5 minutes.

PER 4-OUNCE SERVING: 8g protein, 2g carbohydrates, 7g fat, 1g saturated fat, 71mg sodium, 5mg potassium, 0g fiber

Instant Pot instructions:

1 Follow Steps 1 and 2 of the slow-cooker instructions. Select Sauté (normal heat), add the oil to the Instant Pot and sear the beef for 2 minutes per side. Press Cancel.

2 Stir in the remaining ingredients. Secure the lid.

3 Select Pressure Cook at high pressure for 25 minutes.

4 Use a natural pressure release (about 45 minutes).

5 Transfer the beef to a large bowl and shred with two forks. Discard the bay leaves.

6 Select Sauté (normal heat), bring the sauce to a boil, and reduce, stirring frequently so it doesn't burn.

Dutch-oven instructions (stovetop and oven):

1 Do the math to calculate your braising time before you throw out the meat packaging: weight of roast in pounds × 75 will equal braising time in oven. For example, a 2.06-pound roast would braise for 155 minutes.

2 Preheat oven to 325°F (165°C).

3 Follow Steps 1 to 4 of the slow-cooker instructions.

4 Pour the tomatoes, remaining spice mixture, bay leaves, and 2 cups of water or low-sodium broth over the beef and stir well. Liquid should be at least halfway up the meat, or just covering. Bring to a boil on the stove with the lid on.

5 Place the Dutch oven with the lid on in the oven for time calculated, checking every 90 minutes and flipping the meat over each time. If the liquid starts getting low, add 1–2 cups boiling broth or water. Braise until meat is falling-apart-tender. Discard the 3 bay leaves.

6 Follow Step 8 of the slow-cooker instructions to finish.

COOK'S NOTE: *Use the smaller amount of chipotle powder for a less-spicy version. Thanks to Chef Joann Stabile of Plated with Purpose for sharing her method for this recipe.*

SERVING SUGGESTIONS:
Serve with Chipotle Sweet Potatoes (p. 112) and a green vegetable as sides.

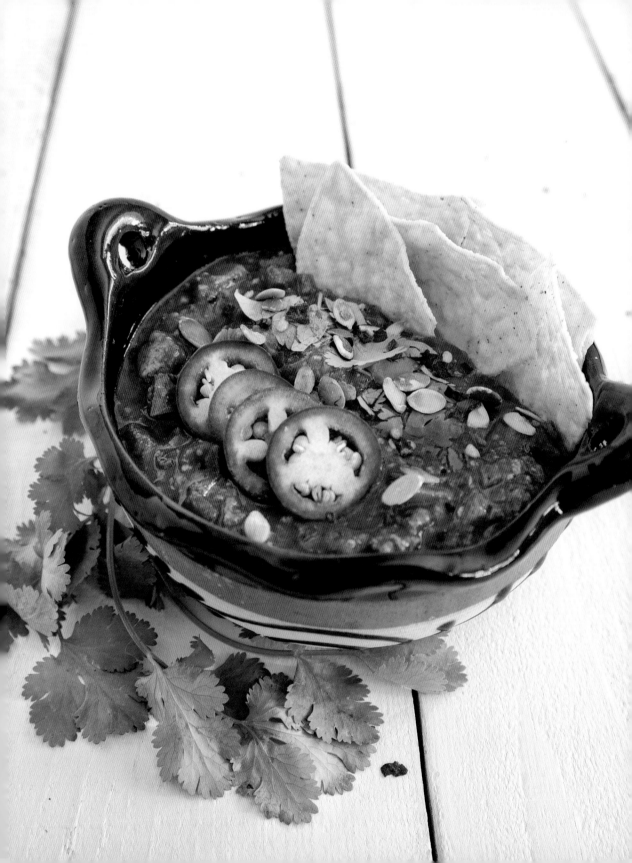

Wild Game Chili

If I eat the same foods week after week, I may not get the variety of nutrients my body may need. For this reason, I try to vary the types of fruits, vegetables, greens, and proteins I eat over the course of a month. Wild game meats are leaner than those raised on factory farms and may contain additional nutrients from the animal's intake. I don't know anyone who hunts, so I buy frozen elk, bison, venison, or wild boar to make this stew. See Cook's Note for other meat substitutions.

Makes 6 servings

Prep time: 20 minutes
Cooking time: 45 minutes
Passive time: N/A

Budget friendly: Moderate

2 tablespoons extra-virgin olive oil

2 carrots, chopped

2 stalks celery, chopped

1 red bell pepper, diced

2 cloves garlic, minced

6 green onions, chopped

1 pound (450g) ground elk, venison, bison, or wild boar

2 tablespoons chili powder

1 teaspoon ground cumin

¼–½ teaspoon chipotle powder or to taste

1 (28-ounce [800g]) can crushed or diced no-salt-added tomatoes

1 (14–15-ounce [410–425g]) can pumpkin or butternut squash puree

Up to 2 cups (500mL) Low-Sodium Vegetable Broth (p. 204) or Low-Sodium Chicken Broth (p. 136), as needed

1 cup (64g) no-salt-added raw or toasted pumpkin seeds

1 teaspoon coconut sugar (optional)

1 Heat the oil over medium heat in a deep skillet or pot with a lid until shimmering. Sauté the carrots, celery, and bell pepper for 5 minutes.

2 Add the garlic and green onions and cook for 1 minute.

3 Add the ground meat and cook until browned and no longer pink, breaking up with a spoon.

4 Stir in the spices and cook 1 more minute.

5 Add the rest of the ingredients and stir well. Add optional broth if mixture seems very thick and dry.

6 Bring just to a boil over high heat, then reduce heat to low and simmer, covered, for at least 30 minutes.

COOK'S NOTE: *You can substitute ground chicken or turkey for the game meat. Ground beef and pork are too fatty for this recipe. Use the smaller amount of chipotle powder if you're sensitive to spice.*

SERVING SUGGESTIONS: Serve over gluten-free rotini or spaghetti for a hearty dinner, or with toasted gluten-free bread.

PER 1-CUP SERVING (with elk and coconut sugar):
25g protein, 17g carbohydrates, 16g fat, 3g saturated fat, 177mg sodium, 559mg potassium, 6g fiber

Chili-Mac Skillet Dinner

When readers requested more quick dinners, I re-engineered a box of "Helper." If you measure and mix the spices while the meat is browning, the entire dish is done in 25 minutes, the same time as the boxed version. Did I mention this includes healthy fats, is low in sodium, and has rich flavor?

Makes 6 servings

Prep time: N/A
Cooking time: 25 minutes
Passive time: N/A

Budget friendly: Very

1 tablespoon extra-virgin olive oil (omit for beef version)

1 pound (450g) ground turkey or grass-fed beef

4 teaspoons cornstarch

1½ tablespoons mild chili powder

2 teaspoons smoked paprika

2 teaspoons coconut sugar (optional)

1 teaspoon ground cumin

1 teaspoon garlic powder

1 teaspoon dried oregano

3 cups (750mL) filtered water

2 tablespoons tomato paste, see Cook's Note

1½ cups (125g) elbow-shape gluten-free pasta

1 Add the oil, if using, to a large skillet on medium-high heat.

2 Add the meat and brown, breaking up with a spoon. Cook until most of the meat is browned. Drain any liquid from the pan.

3 While the meat is cooking, stir the cornstarch and the spices together in a bowl until one color.

4 Heat the water in a saucepan to near boiling.

5 Add the tomato paste to the meat in the pan, then sprinkle the spice mixture over the meat and stir until well combined.

6 Add the uncooked pasta and hot filtered water to the meat pan and stir well. Bring to a boil.

7 Cover and cook for 8 minutes, adjusting the heat so the mixture is bubbling but not a rolling boil. Uncover and cook a few more minutes, until the sauce has thickened and the pasta is tender.

8 Stir in additional ingredients (see Cook's Note) if using.

COOK'S NOTE: *Adding the optional sugar mimics the taste of the boxed version. For best results, find the thinnest gluten-free pasta you can, elbow shape if available. Thicker pasta like rotini or penne will work but requires more cooking time. If you are sensitive to cornstarch, substitute the same amount of tapioca starch. Note that for some recipe testers this yielded 4 servings—maybe because it's so delicious everyone wanted more! Amp up the flavor or extend the dish with any of the following: 1 (15.5-ounce [439g]) can rinsed and drained kidney beans; 1 cup of chopped tomatoes, green onion, and/or bell pepper; 1 minced jalapeño; and/or ½ cup minced cilantro or fresh Italian parsley.*

PER SERVING (⅙ of recipe with ground turkey and coconut sugar):
17g protein, 32g carbohydrates, 9g fat, 2g saturated fat, 47mg sodium, 104mg potassium, 1g fiber

"Resilience to me is to be able to get up every day, no matter what difficulties you're experiencing, and face it. And face it with faith and determination to make the best of it."

KIM CAMPBELL, AUTHOR OF *GENTLE ON MY MIND: IN SICKNESS AND IN HEALTH WITH GLEN CAMPBELL*

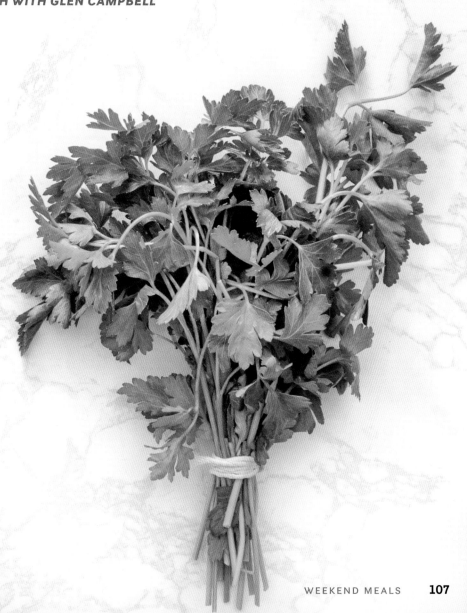

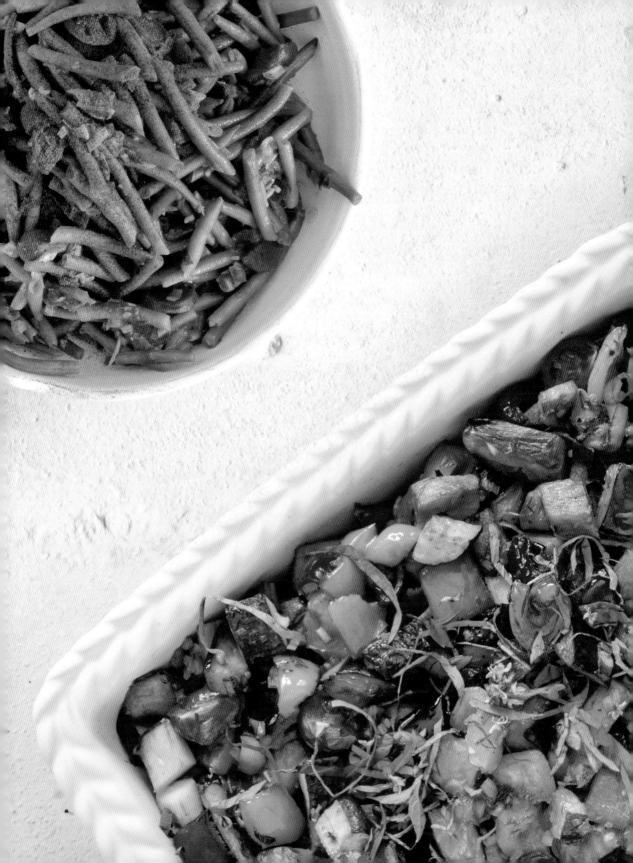

Scrumptious Sides

When I was a vegetarian, I could easily make a meal from small dishes like these. Whether you're eating a plant-based diet or a diet that includes meat, I've provided a variety of ideas for you to choose from. Don't limit these to dinner! Many of these I'd eat for breakfast or lunch.

Coconut-Curried Greens

Healthy fats such as coconut and olive oil bring out the silky texture of dark leafy greens and tame their bitterness. They also make the nutrients in the greens easier for our bodies to absorb. I love the smell of this as it simmers on the stove. It reminds me a bit of sag paneer, a spinach-and-cheese dish served at many Indian restaurants.

Makes 4 servings

Prep time: 10 minutes
Cooking time: 35–65 minutes
Passive time: N/A

Budget friendly: Very

1 tablespoon extra-virgin olive oil or coconut oil

1 tablespoon mild or medium no-salt-added curry powder

2 cloves garlic, minced

1 pound (450g) greens, such as Swiss chard, kale, beet, turnip, or mustard, finely chopped

1 (14-ounce [396g]) can light or regular coconut milk

1 Heat the oil in a cast-iron frying pan or nonstick sauté pan over medium heat until shimmering.

2 Add the curry powder and garlic and cook 1 minute, stirring constantly.

3 Add the greens and cook for about 5 minutes, stirring once or twice, until they start to wilt.

4 Add the coconut milk and stir, mixing thoroughly.

5 Bring just to a boil, then turn down to a simmer, cover, and cook for 30 to 45 minutes, until it looks like a thick sauce.

COOK'S NOTE: *For a creamier texture, pulse the greens in a food processor until finely chopped. If using kale, include the finely chopped stems for extra fiber and potassium. Buy mild curry powder for less spicy results; you'll get all the wonderful flavor and antioxidant benefits without the heat. Spicy-food lovers can top with red chile pepper flakes or hot sauce.*

SERVING SUGGESTIONS: Add leftovers to a breakfast bowl with Easy Roasted Potatoes (p. 148) and an over-easy egg. Pair with South Asian-Inspired Chickpea Masala (p. 86), Curried Roast Cauliflower (p. 115), and Saffron Rice (p. 120).

PER SERVING (with kale and light coconut milk):
3g protein, 16g carbohydrates, 9g fat, 4g saturated fat, 112mg sodium, 535mg potassium, 4g fiber

"Focus on some lifestyle factors that you value anyway, that you think will help you feel better in general and will improve your health and vitality. The hope is that they will also reduce migraine attack frequency. People should choose the things that they're ready to do, that they're excited about, and that they think will help them feel better in general."

**DR. ELIZABETH SENG,
YESHIVA UNIVERSITY**

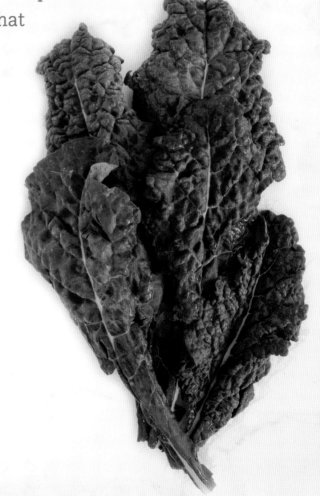

Chipotle Sweet Potatoes

The smoky heat of ground chipotle pepper and some luscious, healthy fat makes these sweet potatoes sing. I love serving this as a side for a holiday meal.

Makes 8 servings

Prep time: 10 minutes
Cooking time: 25 minutes
Passive time: N/A

Budget friendly: Very

2 cups (16 ounces [450g]) sweet potato puree, thawed if frozen

¼ cup (60mL) coconut milk

2 tablespoons ghee or grass-fed butter, melted

½ teaspoon chipotle powder or to taste

1 Preheat oven to 350°F (160°C).

2 Mix all the ingredients together, then spread into an oiled oven-proof casserole dish.

3 Bake 20 to 30 minutes until hot.

COOK'S NOTE: *Use canned or frozen sweet potato puree, or home-roasted sweet potatoes scooped out of the skins. You can substitute canned butternut squash or pumpkin puree, but not pumpkin-pie filling, which contains sugar and spices.*

SERVING SUGGESTIONS: Serve with Beef Barbacoa (p. 102) and a green salad. Excellent with Grilled Salmon, Two Glazes (choose the Smoky Maple topping, p. 65) or Sheet Pan Chicken Thighs (p. 89). See page 208 for a full holiday menu.

PER SERVING: 2g protein, 15g carbohydrates, 5g fat, 4g saturated fat, 47mg sodium, 0mg potassium, 1g fiber

Sweet Potato Oven Fries

If you love fries but want a high-fiber option that's lower on the glycemic index, these should do the trick. Leaving the skins on the sweet potatoes adds nutrition and saves you time.

Makes 4 servings

Prep time:	15 minutes
Cooking time:	25–35 minutes
Passive time:	N/A

Budget friendly: Very

1¾ pounds (800g) sweet potatoes, about 6 medium, cut lengthwise into rustic fries

2 tablespoons extra-virgin olive oil

1 teaspoon garlic powder

½ teaspoon ground cumin

¼ teaspoon cayenne pepper

⅛ teaspoon sea salt (optional)

1 Preheat the oven to 425°F (220°C). Line 2 rimmed baking sheets with parchment paper, non-stick aluminum foil, or silicone sheets. Put the oven rack in the top third of the oven if your heating element is at the bottom of your oven, or in the middle if the heat comes from above.

2 Toss the fries in a large bowl with the olive oil, making sure they are completely coated.

3 Mix the spices together in a small bowl until well incorporated. Sprinkle the spice mixture over the sweet potatoes, stirring and tossing with a large spoon until the fries are evenly coated.

4 Spread the fries onto the prepared sheets, making sure they are not touching each other.

5 Bake for 15 minutes, flip, then bake another 10 to 25 minutes until the fries are browned on the outside and soft inside when pierced with a fork.

COOK'S NOTE: *Use ⅛ teaspoon cayenne if you don't want the fries to be too spicy. If you have smoked salt in the pantry, grind it finely and use instead of sea salt. These won't get as crispy as white potatoes will.*

SERVING SUGGESTIONS: Serve with your favorite mayo as a dipping sauce, such as Cilantro Mayonnaise (p. 268, *The Migraine Relief Plan*), Olive Oil Mayonnaise (p. 195) mixed with Hot Sauce (p. 196), or Chile Pepper Sauce (p. 267, *The Migraine Relief Plan*). They're the perfect side dish for Veggie Burgers (p. 71) or Sheet Pan Chicken Thighs (p. 89).

PER SERVING (with added salt): 3g protein, 40g carbohydrates, 7g fat, 1g saturated fat, 184mg sodium, 674mg potassium, 6g fiber

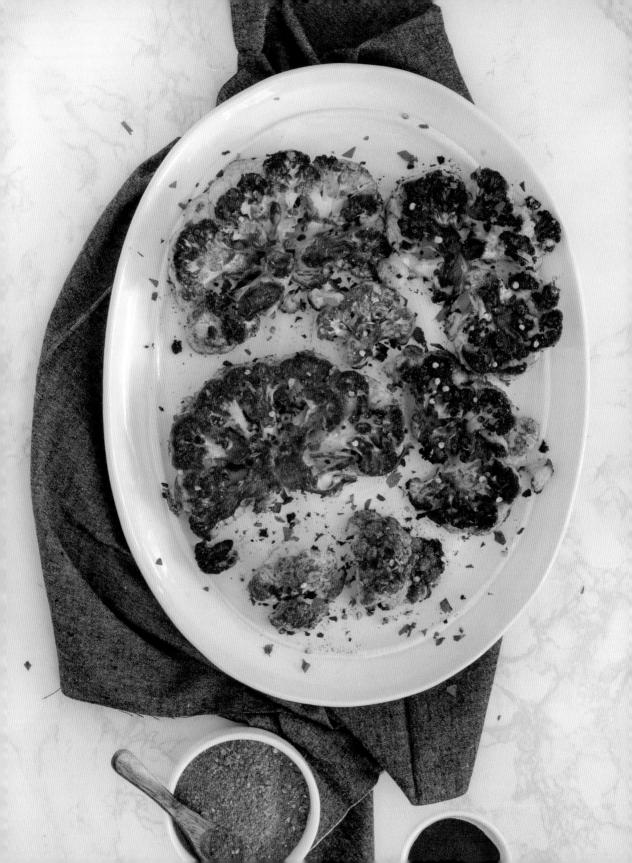

Curried Roast Cauliflower

I thought I hated cauliflower until my neighbor served it as a main dish, roasted at high heat and lightly spiced. Ding! The bitterness and mushy texture were gone, replaced with caramelized, savory edges.

Makes 4 servings

Prep time: 10 minutes
Cooking time: 25–30 minutes
Passive time: N/A

Budget friendly: Very

1 head cauliflower

2 tablespoons extra-virgin olive oil, plus more for oiling pan

1 tablespoon no-salt-added mild curry powder

½ teaspoon smoked paprika

¼ teaspoon chipotle or cayenne powder, or to taste

1 Preheat oven to 450°F (230°C).

2 Wash the cauliflower and shake dry. Remove leaves and cut out core.

3 Cut cauliflower vertically into slices ½-inch (1.25cm) thick.

4 In a large bowl, whisk together the oil, curry powder, smoked paprika, and chipotle or cayenne powder.

5 Add the cauliflower slices and toss to coat until evenly colored with spice mixture. Spread in a single layer in a large oiled baking pan.

6 Bake until the cauliflower is tender, chewy, and brown, 25 to 30 minutes, flipping halfway through.

COOK'S NOTE: *If you don't like curry powder, substitute 1 teaspoon of dried cumin.*

SERVING SUGGESTIONS: Serve with Coconut-Curried Greens (p. 110) and roasted meat or Grilled Salmon, Two Glazes (p. 65).

PER SERVING: 3g protein, 7g carbohydrates, 7g fat, 1g saturated fat, 0mg sodium, 628mg potassium, 3g fiber

Green Bean Casserole

I "renovated" the holiday classic without the fried onions and high-sodium cream of mushroom soup so you can still enjoy it with your family. Is it slightly different? Yes. Might you like it better? Possibly.

Makes 8 servings

Prep time: 20 minutes
Cooking time: 35 minutes
Passive time: N/A

Budget friendly: Moderate

1 ¼ teaspoons sea salt, divided

1 pound (450g) green beans, fresh or frozen and thawed, see Cook's Note

½ cup (125mL) whole, hemp, or light coconut milk

1 cup (250mL) Rich Mushroom Gravy (p. 206)

½ cup (60g) toasted sunflower seeds

¼ cup (15g) freeze-dried shallots, see Cook's Note

1 Preheat oven to 350°F (160°C).

2 Bring a large pot of filtered water to a boil and add 1 teaspoon of the sea salt. Add the beans to the boiling water and cook for 4 minutes. Drain well in a colander, rinsing with cold water.

3 In a small bowl, stir the milk into the gravy, mixing until smooth.

4 Put the sunflower seeds in a food processor and pulse until you have large crumbs. Add the shallots and the remaining ¼ teaspoon of salt and pulse just until broken up.

5 Spray or oil a large baking dish and add the beans. Pour the gravy mixture over the beans and stir to coat evenly. Sprinkle the sunflower seed mixture evenly over the top.

6 Bake for 30 minutes, until the top is lightly browned and the casserole is bubbly. Serve immediately.

COOK'S NOTE: *Prepare fresh green beans by washing and draining them well. Cut off the stems and tips and slice them into 3-inch (10cm) pieces. If you like your beans firm, skip Step 2. Freeze- or air-dried shallots are available from Penzeys and stand in for the fried onions that typically top this dish.*

SERVING SUGGESTIONS: See my full Holiday Menu on page 208.

PER SERVING (with hemp milk): 4g protein, 8g carbohydrates, 5g fat, 1g saturated fat, 153mg sodium, 325mg potassium, 2g fiber

Garlic Mashed Potatoes

Have I already mentioned I could live on potatoes alone? Adding garlic powder helps replace the level of salt you might be used to without sacrificing flavor. Yes, you can eat favorite foods like mashed potatoes on the Plan. I'm not a monster! This is an easy side dish for a weeknight.

Makes 8 servings

Prep time: 20 minutes
Cooking time: 35 minutes
Passive time: N/A

Budget friendly: Very

1 pound (450g) gold or red potatoes, quartered

1½ teaspoons granulated garlic or garlic powder

½ teaspoon freshly ground black pepper

¼ teaspoon sea salt

Up to 1 cup (250mL) whole, hemp, or light coconut milk, warmed

1 Bring a large pot of filtered water to a boil.

2 Add the potatoes to the boiling water and cook for 10 to 25 minutes until they pierce easily with a fork. Drain well in a colander.

3 Return the potatoes to the pot with the seasonings and begin mashing, using a potato masher or ricer. Add milk as needed to get the consistency you like. Serve immediately.

COOK'S NOTE: *Choose organic potatoes if you can find them. I prefer gold potatoes, which have a delightfully creamy texture even before mashing. Leave the skins on unless you notice the potatoes have a green tinge. If you prefer a whipped texture, use an electric hand mixer or potato masher. Don't use a food processor or blender, or the potatoes will be gummy. Fresh or dried chives, dried parsley, smoked paprika, and butter can be added for more flavor.*

SERVING SUGGESTIONS: See my full Holiday Menu on page 208. Great with Roasted Chicken with Veggie Gravy (p. 134).

PER SERVING (with hemp milk): 2g protein, 10g carbohydrates, 3g fat, 0g saturated fat, 121mg sodium, 234mg potassium, 1g fiber

Lebanese Green Beans

I enjoyed this dish at a Lebanese restaurant in Paris after we visited the Louvre. It was so delightful and different than any other green bean dish I'd ever had, I asked the owner to explain it to me, despite my limited French. Don't skip the cinnamon; it's one of the things that makes the flavor special.

Makes 4 servings

Prep time: 15–20 minutes
Cooking time: 15–25 minutes
Passive time: N/A

Budget friendly: Very

1 tablespoon extra-virgin olive oil

6 green onions, thinly sliced

3 cloves garlic, finely minced

8 ounces (225g) fresh tomatoes, cored and chopped, or no-salt-added canned

¼ teaspoon white pepper

¼ teaspoon freshly ground black pepper

⅛ teaspoon cinnamon

1 pound (450g) green beans (French *haricots verts* if available), ends trimmed, sliced on the diagonal into 2-inch pieces

1 Heat the oil in a large sauté pan or Dutch oven over medium-high heat. When the oil is hot, add the green onions.

2 Sauté for 1 minute and then reduce the heat to medium. Add the garlic and sauté for about 6 minutes, stirring regularly and reducing the heat if necessary.

3 Add the tomatoes and spices and cook 5 minutes.

4 Add the beans. If using thin *haricots verts*, cook about 3 minutes. Regular green beans need to cook longer: Test them after 8 minutes. Beans should be softened but not mushy.

5 Serve the beans hot, cold, or room temperature. They're even better the next day after the flavors have developed.

COOK'S NOTE: Haricots verts *are very thin and cook quickly. If you substitute frozen green beans (either regular or thin), thaw before using.*

SERVING SUGGESTIONS: See my full Summer BBQ menu on page 209.

PER SERVING: 3g protein, 13g carbohydrates, 4g fat, 1g saturated fat, 17mg sodium, 409mg potassium, 5g fiber

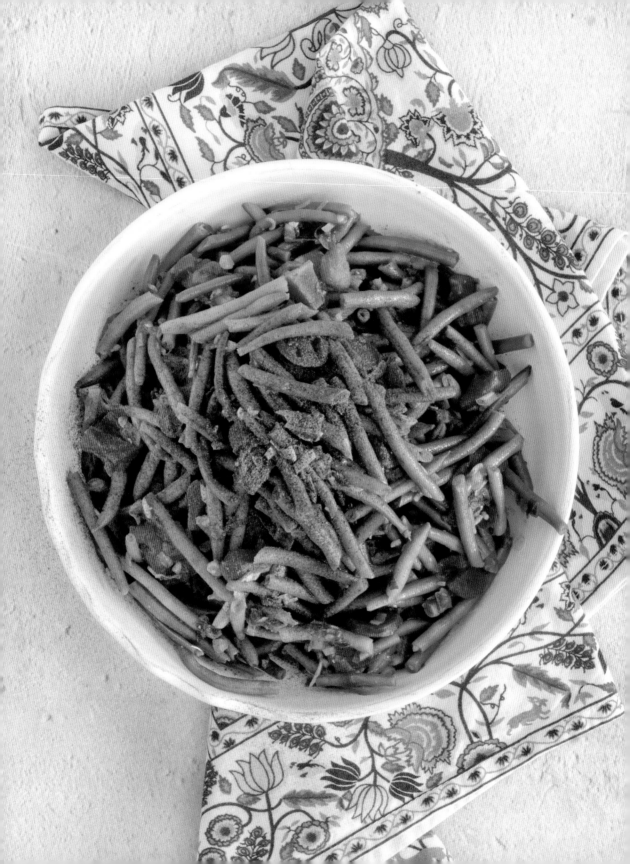

Saffron Rice

While saffron is expensive, you only need a tiny amount for this recipe. It adds gorgeous color and subtle flavor. Persian, Kashmiri, and Spanish saffron vary in intensity and flavor.

Makes 8 servings

Prep time: 5 minutes
Cooking time: 15 minutes
Passive time: 15 minutes

Budget friendly: Moderate

3 cups (750mL) filtered or spring water

½ teaspoon saffron threads (see Cook's Note)

1½ cups (270g) white basmati or jasmine rice, rinsed and drained 6 times until water runs clear

1 Heat the water in a medium-size saucepan until hot but not boiling. Remove from heat and add the saffron. Let it steep with the lid on for at least 15 minutes.

2 When you are 20 minutes from meal time, bring the saffron-infused water to a boil. Add the rice, cover, turn heat to low, and cook 10 to 12 minutes. Turn heat off and let sit with the lid on until you are ready to serve. Fluff gently with a fork.

COOK'S NOTE: *One teaspoon of turmeric can be substituted for the saffron; skip Step 1. Brown basmati or jasmine rice will also work, but not short-grain styles such as sushi rice. Adjust cooking time accordingly based on package instructions.*

SERVING SUGGESTIONS: Excellent with seafood, like a delicate shrimp dish or my Thai-Style Shrimp Curry (p. 153), or Fish Baked in Parchment Packets (p. 228, *The Migraine Relief Plan*). Try it with South Asian-Inspired Chickpea Masala (p. 86), Sheet Pan Chicken Thighs (p. 89), or chicken cooked with Pomegranate Marinade (p. 270, *The Migraine Relief Plan*).

PER SERVING: 2g protein, 27g carbohydrates, 0g fat, 0g saturated fat, 0mg sodium, 0mg potassium, 1g fiber

Pumpkin Risotto

This recipe marries the concept of Italian risotto with non-traditional ingredients for a creamy dish with no dairy added. If you've never made risotto, don't be intimidated; it just takes a little patience and some stirring. If I needed to bring a side to a holiday meal, this one is guaranteed to surprise the other guests, with the combination of pumpkin, ginger, and garam masala.

Makes 6 servings

Prep time:　　　10 minutes
Cooking time:　45 minutes
Passive time:　N/A

Budget friendly: Moderate

4 ½ cups (1.25L) Low-Sodium Vegetable Broth (p. 204) or Low-Sodium Chicken Broth (p. 136)

1 tablespoon extra-virgin olive oil

1 shallot, minced

2 cloves garlic, minced

1-inch piece of fresh ginger root (10g), minced

1 teaspoon garam masala, either a no-salt-added store-bought version or mine (p. 199)

1 teaspoon smoked paprika

1 cup (235g) Arborio rice

1 (15-ounce [425g]) can pumpkin puree

1 Heat the broth in a saucepan on medium heat until simmering, then maintain a very low simmer as you continue with the following steps.

2 Heat the oil in a large sauté pan over medium heat and add the shallot. Fry for 3 minutes, then add the garlic, ginger, garam masala, and paprika and fry 2 minutes more.

3 Add the rice and cook, stirring, about 2 minutes.

4 Ladle in about ½ cup of the hot broth and use a wooden spoon to scrape up any burnt bits from the bottom of the pan. Stir almost constantly until all the liquid is absorbed, then add another ladle full of broth. It should take 7 to 8 minutes to absorb about a cup of liquid. If it is taking a lot longer, raise the heat just a little. If it is taking much less time, reduce the heat a little.

5 After about 30 minutes, when you have about a cup of broth left to add, add in the pumpkin and remaining broth. Continue cooking and stirring on low, uncovered, until the rice is tender. It should still have a loose texture.

COOK'S NOTE: *If you wish to use fresh pumpkin, roast 1 small pie pumpkin (350 to 450g). The pumpkin should be roasted until tender, then peeled and minced. Add 1 to 2 cups to this recipe in Step 5 in place of the pumpkin puree. Italian risotto would be cooked in Step 5 until al dente (having a slight bite to it). I prefer my rice a bit more tender.*

SERVING SUGGESTIONS: Serve with South Asian-Inspired Chickpea Masala (p. 86) and Coconut-Curried Greens (p. 110). Or include in a Holiday Menu (p. 208).

PER SERVING: 3g protein, 21g carbohydrates, 3g fat, 0g saturated fat, 54mg sodium, 12mg potassium, 2g fiber

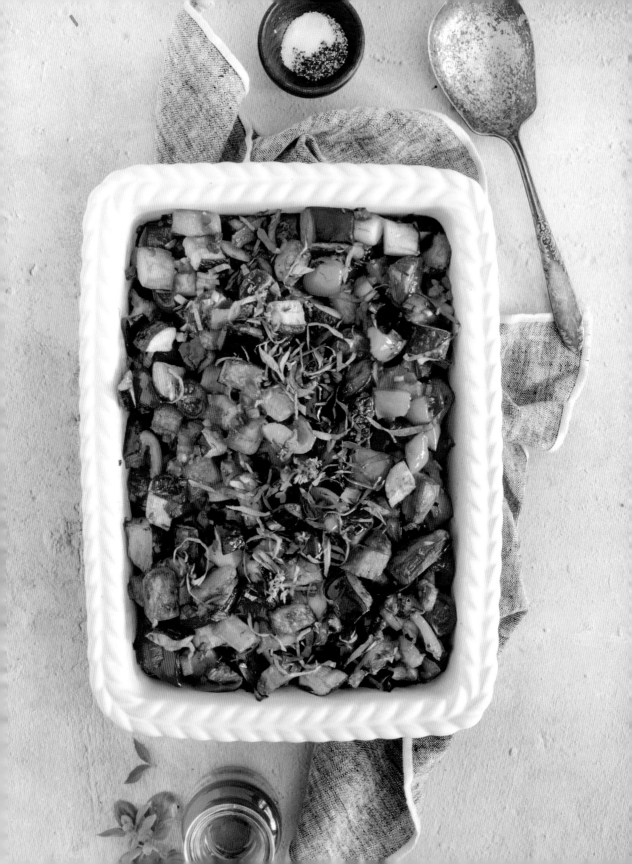

Ratatouille

This beautiful Provençal dish uses up the bounty of a summer garden. I had a memorable version on my 50th birthday at my friend's home in Tarascon, a small town in Southern France. Don't skimp on the olive oil, it's what adds the rich flavor.

Makes 8 servings

Prep time: 30 minutes
Cooking time: 1 hour
              15 minutes
Passive time: N/A

Budget friendly: Very

4 tablespoons extra-virgin olive oil, divided

12 green onions, thinly sliced

4 cloves garlic, thinly sliced

2 eggplants, diced medium

2 zucchinis, diced medium

2 red or yellow bell peppers, seeded and cut into chunks

4 plum or 8–12 cherry tomatoes, diced

2–3 sprigs fresh thyme

1 handful fresh basil leaves

1 Preheat oven to 350°F (180°C).

2 Heat 1 tablespoon of the olive oil in a large cast-iron or nonstick pan over medium-high heat. Sauté the green onions until they are soft.

3 Add the garlic and cook until soft.

4 Transfer to a deep roasting pan or oven-safe baking dish, leaving the pan on the stove.

5 Sauté the eggplant, zucchini, and peppers separately, adding more oil as needed, until each is golden. Transfer each to the baking dish as it is finished.

6 Stir the diced tomatoes and thyme into the baking dish, seasoning with a tiny amount of salt and a generous amount of black pepper. Drizzle with additional olive oil.

7 Bake for about 40 minutes until soft and tender.

8 Discard the thyme stems and stir in a handful of torn basil leaves before serving.

COOK'S NOTE: *If you have them, add one sprig of fresh rosemary and a few sprigs of fresh oregano to the ratatouille in Step 6.*

SERVING SUGGESTIONS: Serve over warm spaghetti squash strands, which can be baked at the same time as the ratatouille. For a Mediterranean-inspired meal, pair with any of these dishes: Lebanese Green Beans (p. 118), Pan-Roasted Kale with Crispy Italian Breadcrumbs (p. 129), Mediterranean Tuna Burgers (p. 70), Provençal Chickpea Salad (p. 218, *The Migraine Relief Plan*), Tuscan White Bean Soup (p. 144), or Pasta e Fagioli (p. 145).

PER SERVING: 7g protein, 25g carbohydrates, 8g fat, 1g saturated fat, 34mg sodium, 1032mg potassium, 10g fiber

Roasted Garlic-Jalapeño Grits

I first tasted this dish at the Hawaii Food and Wine Festival in Honolulu. I loved it so much I asked the chef for the recipe and adapted it for the Plan. It is very hearty paired with poached eggs.

Makes 4 servings

Prep time: 5 minutes
Cooking time: 25 minutes
Passive time: N/A

Budget friendly: Very

1 cup (135g) stone-ground white corn grits or stone-ground polenta

2 teaspoons garlic powder

¼ teaspoon sea salt (optional)

1–2 jalapeño peppers (or to taste), stemmed and seeded

3 tablespoons heavy cream or full-fat coconut milk

½ teaspoon freshly ground black pepper

1 Heat 4 cups (.95L) of filtered water in a large heavy-bottomed pot over high heat until boiling. Slowly pour in the grits while whisking constantly. Whisk in the garlic powder and sea salt if using. Reduce the heat to low, cover, and cook for about 20 minutes, stirring occasionally.

2 While the grits are cooking, turn on the broiler. Press the pepper, skin side up, onto a piece of heavy aluminum foil, and broil until the entire skin is black and blistered. Using tongs, drop it into a paper bag, close the bag, and let cool. When the pepper is cool enough to handle, remove and discard the skin.

3 Mince the pepper and add it to the pot of grits.

4 Remove the pot from the heat and whisk thoroughly. Stir in the cream or milk and pepper. Taste and season with additional black pepper if needed.

COOK'S NOTE: *If you do not like spicy food, choose a mild pepper for roasting. You can use a gas burner or a dry skillet on high heat to roast the pepper. Substitute canned, diced green chiles if the brand is Plan-friendly. You can roast 3 unpeeled cloves of garlic with the peppers, then let cool and squeeze them into the grits instead of the garlic powder. If you can tolerate salt, it really enhances the flavor of the grits.*

SERVING SUGGESTIONS: Serve as the base for poached eggs with some steamed spinach, with pan-seared shrimp for a quick shrimp and grits, or with Pan-Roasted Kale with Crispy Italian Breadcrumbs (p. 129) and beef slow cooked in Pomegranate Marinade (p. 270, *The Migraine Relief Plan*).

PER SERVING (without added salt): 3g protein, 29g carbohydrates, 4g fat, 3g saturated fat, 8mg sodium, 60mg potassium, 2g fiber

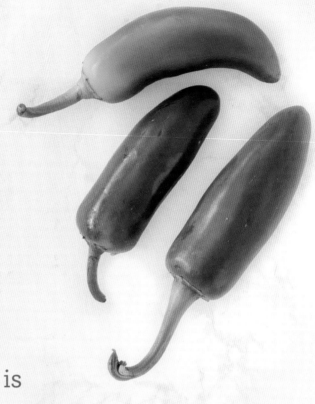

"Migraine disease is
absolutely not something
that is wrong with you as a
person. It's not a weakness.
I learned cognitive behavioral
therapy and mindfulness. I
have those techniques that
I turn to when things are
particularly difficult."

**DR. JENNIFER ROBBLEE,
BARROW NEUROLOGICAL INSTITUTE**

Oven-Roasted Vegetables with Greek Spice Blend

I was given a delicious spice blend by a Greek olive-oil importer, and I loved how it enhances the caramelized flavor of roasted vegetables. So I created a no-salt-added version for this recipe.

Makes 8 servings

Prep time: 10 minutes
Cooking time: 25-30 minutes
Passive time: N/A

Budget friendly: Very

2 tablespoons extra-virgin olive oil

2 pounds (900g) organic gold or red new potatoes (approximately 8 small potatoes), cut into 2-inch chunks

4 carrots, cut into 1½-inch pieces

1 teaspoon Greek Spice Blend (p. 200)

1 Preheat oven to 450°F (230°C). Toss the vegetables with the oil on a rimmed baking sheet, leaving space between them. Sprinkle evenly with the Greek Spice Blend.

2 Roast the vegetables for 25 to 30 minutes, turning after 15 minutes. Check with a fork and remove when fork tender. Outsides should be golden brown and crispy. Serve immediately or at room temperature.

COOK'S NOTE: *It's important to cut the vegetables into same-size pieces so they cook uniformly. Very small potatoes can be roasted whole. Other vegetables to try include peeled butternut squash, delicata squash, turnips, rutabagas, parsnips, and sweet potatoes. Add more olive oil and spice blend as needed. When roasting a lot of vegetables, I place one type of vegetable on each sheet, as they cook at different speeds.*

SERVING SUGGESTIONS: Serve with Pan-Roasted Kale with Crispy Italian Breadcrumbs (p. 129), Roasted Chicken with Veggie Gravy (p. 134), Lazy Chicken (p. 90), Sheet Pan Chicken Thighs (p. 89), Grilled Salmon, Two Glazes (p. 65), Beef Barbacoa (p. 102), or Fish Baked in Parchment Packets (p. 228, *The Migraine Relief Plan*).

PER SERVING: 0g protein, 24g carbohydrates, 3g fat, 0g saturated fat, 25mg sodium, 590mg potassium, 3g fiber

Stuffed Acorn Squash

This beautiful side makes a wonderful addition to a holiday table (just double or triple the recipe) and can easily be a plant-based main dish without the cheese. Testers raved about this one.

Makes 2–4 servings

Prep time: 30 minutes
Cooking time: 90 minutes
Passive time: N/A

Budget friendly: Moderate

1 acorn squash, ends trimmed, sliced in half across the middle, seeds set aside in a pot of filtered water

1 cup (250mL) filtered water

½ cup (90g) red or tan quinoa, rinsed and drained

1 cup (250mL) Low-Sodium Vegetable Broth (p. 204) or Low-Sodium Chicken Broth (p. 136)

2 small (100g) persimmons, cored and diced

½ cup (65g) chopped Swiss chard, any color

¼ cup (30g) raw, shelled pumpkin seeds

½ cup (130g) ricotta cheese (optional)

½ teaspoon dried sage

¼ teaspoon chipotle powder

¼ teaspoon ground cumin

¼ teaspoon white pepper

1 tablespoon extra-virgin olive oil

1 teaspoon smoked paprika

¼ teaspoon sea salt

1 Preheat the oven to 350°F (160°C).

2 Place the squash cut-side down in an oiled baking pan. Bake 30 to 40 minutes or until soft. Leave the oven on.

3 Rinse the squash seeds. In a saucepan, bring the water and seeds to a boil, then simmer for 10 minutes. Drain and set aside.

4 Add the quinoa to the broth in a saucepan. Bring to a boil, then turn down and simmer for 15 minutes on low. Turn off and let sit for at least 5 minutes, then fluff with a fork.

5 Mix the cooked quinoa, persimmons, chard, pumpkin seeds, cheese (if using), and spices in a large bowl.

6 Once the squash is cooked, carefully scoop out most of the flesh into the quinoa mixture, leaving ½ inch inside. Be careful not to poke through the skin. Mash the squash evenly into the filling, then taste and adjust seasoning if needed. Pack the filling into the squash halves and return to the baking pan.

7 Put the rinsed squash seeds in one corner of the baking pan, adding the olive oil, paprika, and salt. Stir to coat the seeds, then spread into a single layer.

8 Bake for 30 to 45 minutes until the filling is hot. Top squash halves with the toasted squash seeds and a drizzle of olive oil.

COOK'S NOTE: *If you can't find persimmons, use one firm pear. Swiss chard may also be labeled green chard. This filling does not work well with butternut squash; be sure to use acorn or a small spaghetti squash. One tester substituted fresh chèvre for the ricotta and loved the result. If you have fresh sage, use 3 minced leaves in place of the dried sage. You can skip preparing the squash seeds, although most testers loved the texture they added to the finished dish.*

SERVING SUGGESTIONS: Serve as a one-dish vegetarian or plant-based meal. Thrill vegetarian or vegan guests by preparing it as their main course for a Holiday Menu (p. 208).

PER ¼-SQUASH SERVING (with low-sodium vegetable broth and whole-milk ricotta): 1
1g protein, 58g carbohydrates, 8g fat, 3g saturated fat, 129mg sodium, 769mg potassium, 8g fiber

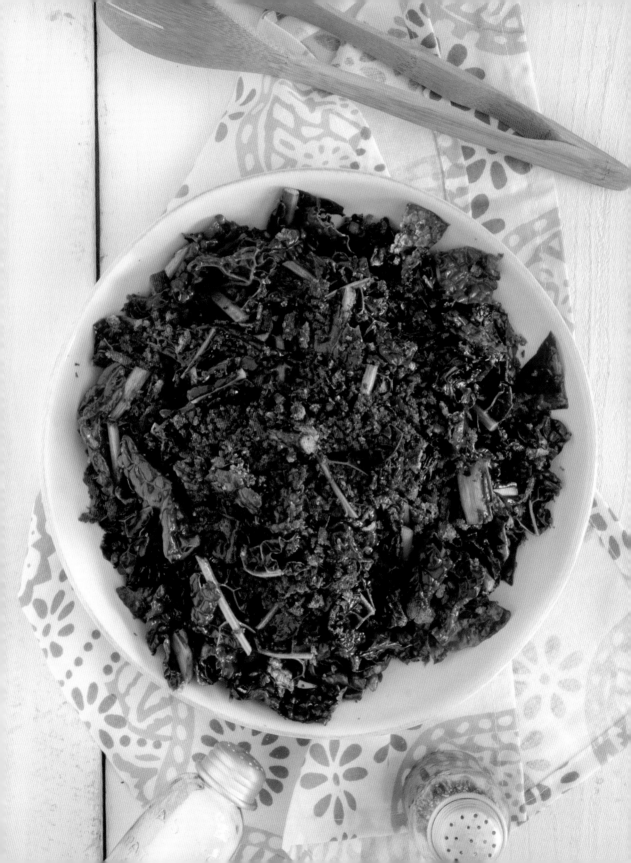

Pan-Roasted Kale with
Crispy Italian Breadcrumbs

This dish was inspired by a favorite side at a restaurant called True Food Kitchen.

Makes 4 servings

Prep time: 10 minutes
Cooking time: 10 minutes
Passive time: N/A

Budget friendly: Very

1 pound (450g) Tuscan or Lacinato kale, roughly chopped

4–6 pieces gluten-free bread, toasted, or 1 cup (120g) gluten-free panko or breadcrumbs

1 tablespoon no-salt-added Italian seasoning blend

2 tablespoons extra-virgin olive oil, divided

1 Finely chop or pulse the toasted bread in a food processor to make breadcrumbs. Add the Italian seasoning and stir to combine.

2 Heat 1 tablespoon of the oil over medium heat in a nonstick or cast-iron pan, swirling to coat.

3 When the oil is shimmering, add the breadcrumbs and sauté until crispy. Pour out onto a plate. Do not wipe out the pan.

4 Add the remaining 1 tablespoon of oil and wait until it shimmers. Add the kale and sauté for 8 to 10 minutes, until wilted and crispy in spots. If the kale gets dry, add a couple tablespoons of low-sodium broth.

5 Top with the breadcrumbs and serve immediately.

COOK'S NOTE: *I freeze the heels of gluten-free loaves for this recipe. Rendered bacon fat from Make Your Own Bacon (p. 197, The Migraine Relief Plan) is wonderful in place of the oil in this dish. I recommend using Lacinato kale (also known as Tuscan or dinosaur) for best results, and because the stems are more tender than those of curly kale, you can include them. If using curly kale, remove the stems, thinly slice, and freeze them to use in Breakfast Hash (p. 38). Curly kale may need to be cooked longer in Step 4.*

SERVING SUGGESTIONS: Serve with Oven-Roasted Vegetables with Greek Spice Blend (p. 126), Ratatouille (p. 123), Roasted Chicken with Veggie Gravy (p. 134), Lazy Chicken (p. 90), Sheet Pan Chicken Thighs (p. 89), Grilled Salmon, Two Glazes (p. 65), Beef Barbacoa (p. 102), pasta topped with Chunky Tomato Sauce (p. 188), Chicken Cacciatore (p. 226, *The Migraine Relief Plan*), Fish Baked in Parchment Packets (p. 228, *The Migraine Relief Plan*), or Meatloaf (p. 230, *The Migraine Relief Plan*).

PER SERVING (with 4 slices Trader Joe's Gluten Free Multigrain Brown Rice Bread):
5g protein, 28g carbohydrates, 10g fat, 1g saturated fat, 154mg sodium, 510mg potassium, 3g fiber

Wild Rice Stuffing

I've made a version of this stuffing for over 30 years. It's that good. I could happily eat this with Rich Mushroom Gravy (p. 206) for my entire holiday meal.

Makes 12 servings

Prep time:	30 minutes
Cooking time:	2 hours
Passive time:	N/A

Budget friendly: Very

1 cup (160g) wild rice, rinsed well

2 cups (500mL) filtered water

2 tablespoons extra-virgin olive oil

4 stalks celery, thinly sliced

12 green onions, thinly sliced

8 ounces (225g) cremini or button mushrooms, thinly sliced

1½ teaspoons dried thyme, crushed

1½ teaspoons dried rosemary, crushed

1½ teaspoons freshly ground black pepper

12 slices gluten-free bread, diced (½–¾-inch)

2 large apples, cored and diced (½–¾-inch)

Up to 4 cups (.95L) Low-Sodium Vegetable Broth (p. 204) or Low-Sodium Chicken Broth (p. 136)

1 Bring the wild rice and water to a boil in a saucepan, then cover and simmer for 45 to 50 minutes until tender. Drain excess water, then set aside and let cool.

2 Preheat the oven to 350°F (180°C). Spray or oil a 9 × 13-inch (23 × 33cm) baking pan.

3 Heat the olive oil in a large sauté pan over medium-high heat until shimmering. Swirl pan to coat. Sauté the celery, onions, mushrooms, herbs, and spices for about 15 minutes, until they are golden brown, and all moisture has evaporated from the pan.

4 In a large bowl, combine the wild rice and vegetable mixture with the remaining ingredients, adding just enough vegetable or chicken broth to moisten the bread without it becoming soggy. Spread stuffing into the baking dish.

5 Bake for 35 to 45 minutes until golden brown on top. Leftover stuffing can be frozen.

COOK'S NOTE: *The wild rice and the vegetable mixture can each be cooked a day in advance. Rome Beauty or Honeycrisp apples are recommended for this recipe. This recipe is egg-free if your gluten-free bread doesn't contain eggs. Use any type of gluten-free bread that's Plan-friendly. If you use a smaller, deeper baking dish, you may need to bake this for 50 to 55 minutes.*

SERVING SUGGESTIONS: Serve as part of a Holiday Menu (p. 208). Delicious with Rich Mushroom Gravy (p. 206), or Roasted Chicken with Veggie Gravy (p. 134).

PER SERVING (with low-sodium vegetable broth and Trader Joe's Gluten Free Multigrain Brown Rice Bread):
6g protein, 37g carbohydrates, 5g fat, 0g saturated fat, 119mg sodium, 445mg potassium, 4g fiber

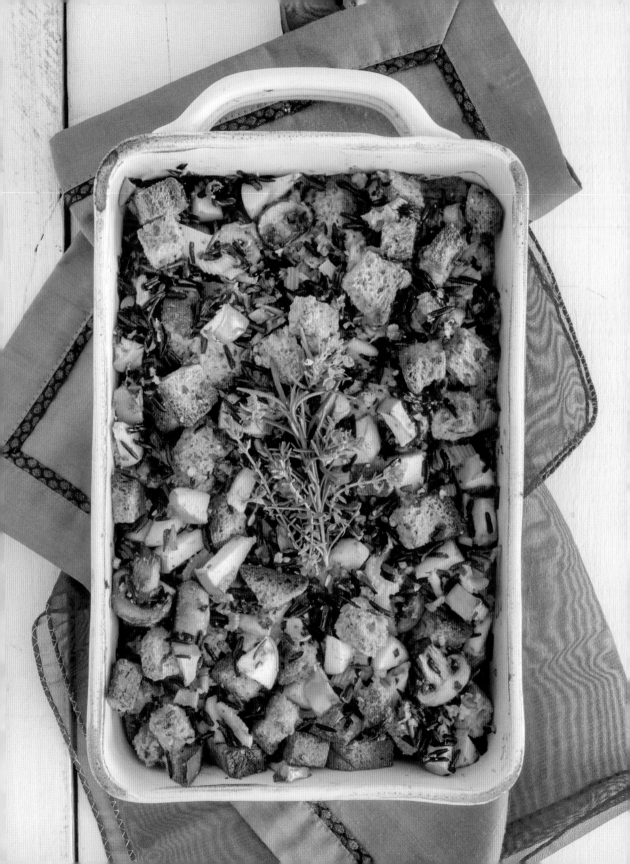

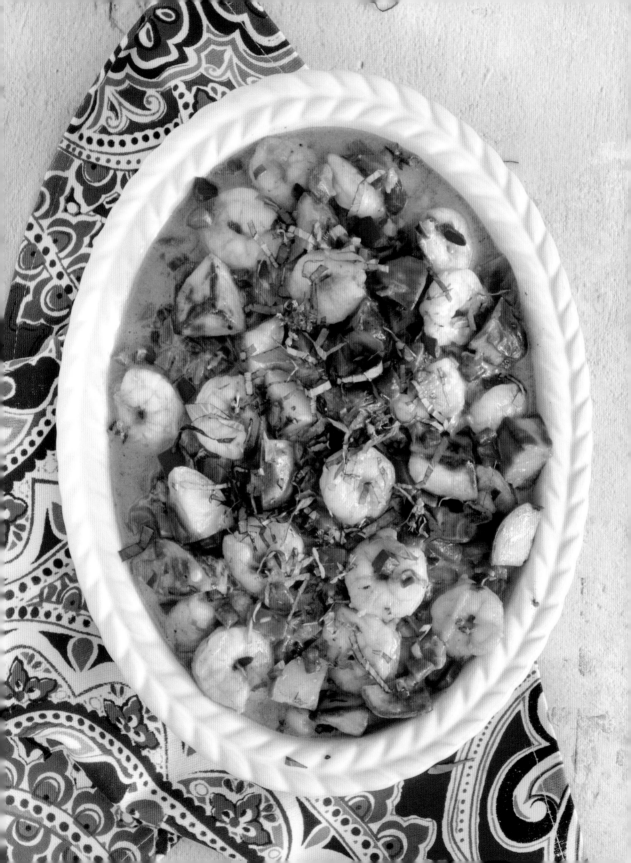

Progressive Cooking

My favorite chapter of *The Migraine Relief Plan* is called Recipes that Use Leftovers. Readers have told me it was quite helpful to them in understanding better ways to use up what they have. In that spirit, I created three base recipes for this book and then several recipes you can make using those leftovers.

Roasted Chicken with Veggie Gravy

Once you learn how to roast a chicken, you may never buy a rotisserie bird again, especially since those are high in sodium. With this recipe, not only do you end up with outstanding gravy, you will be able to use leftovers in the dishes that follow, and even make a delicious broth from the bones.

Makes 8 servings

Prep time: 15 minutes
Cooking time: 2 hours
Passive time: N/A

Budget friendly: Very

3 tablespoons extra-virgin olive oil, divided

4–6 carrots, diced small

6 green onions, thinly sliced

4–6 stalks celery, diced small

1 roasting chicken, patted dry (see Cook's Note)

1 teaspoon freshly ground black pepper

½ teaspoon sea salt (optional)

2 cups (475mL) Low-Sodium Chicken Broth (p. 136), divided

¼ cup (40g) brown rice flour

SERVING SUGGESTIONS:
Delicious with Easy Roasted Potatoes (p. 148), Pan-Roasted Kale with Crispy Italian Breadcrumbs (p. 129), and Spicy Kale and Swiss Chard Sauté (p. 243, *The Migraine Relief Plan*).

1 Preheat oven to 425°F (220°C).

2 Determine roasting time by multiplying the weight of the chicken (in pounds) by 15. For example, a 5.65-pound chicken would roast for 85 minutes.

3 Drizzle 2 tablespoons of the olive oil over the vegetables in a large roasting pan and toss to coat.

4 Drizzle the remaining 1 tablespoon olive oil over the chicken and sprinkle generously with the black pepper and sea salt (if using). Massage the oil into the chicken skin until evenly coated.

5 Place the chicken, breast side up, on top of the vegetables and cook for the time determined in Step 2. When fully cooked, chicken should read 165°F (74°C) on an instant-read thermometer stuck into the thickest part of the thigh.

6 Transfer the chicken to a cutting board to rest while making the gravy.

7 If your roasting pan can go directly on the stove (for instance, a stainless-steel pan), set it on a burner (or burners) on medium heat and skip to Step 8. If not, place it on the stove without heat underneath and pour ¼ cup of the chicken broth into the pan. Using a wooden spoon, scrape and loosen all the brown bits beneath the vegetables in the roasting pan, then pour everything into a sauté or saucepan set on medium heat.

8 Sprinkle the flour over the roasted vegetables and cook, stirring, until flour darkens to golden brown, about 5 to 8 minutes.

9 Slowly add the remaining chicken broth and continue stirring and cooking until the gravy thickens, at least 5 minutes more.

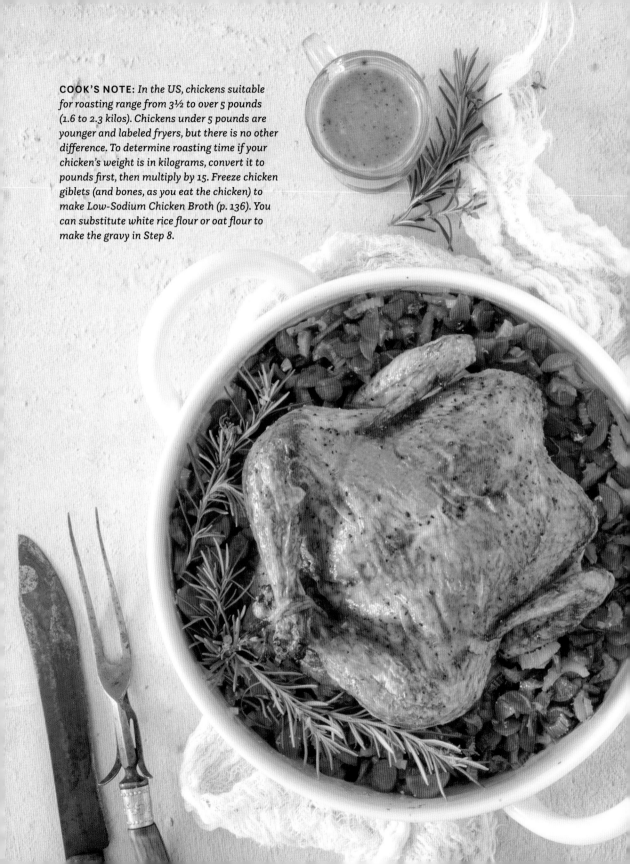

COOK'S NOTE: *In the US, chickens suitable for roasting range from 3½ to over 5 pounds (1.6 to 2.3 kilos). Chickens under 5 pounds are younger and labeled fryers, but there is no other difference. To determine roasting time if your chicken's weight is in kilograms, convert it to pounds first, then multiply by 15. Freeze chicken giblets (and bones, as you eat the chicken) to make Low-Sodium Chicken Broth (p. 136). You can substitute white rice flour or oat flour to make the gravy in Step 8.*

Low-Sodium Chicken Broth

This is the base for so many recipes, and it's crazy-easy to make. Plus, it shows respect for the chickens when we utilize every bit of nutrition they provide for us. Start with the bones from leftover Roasted Chicken with Veggie Gravy.

Makes 12–16 servings

Prep time: 5 minutes
Cooking time: 2-48 hours
Passive time: N/A

Budget friendly: Very

Leftover bones from 1 or more chickens

6 chicken feet or necks (optional)

Green tops from green onions and leeks (whatever you have)

3 bay leaves

2 tablespoons white or apple cider vinegar

16 cups (4L) filtered water

 If apple cider vinegar is not a trigger for you, use in place of white vinegar.

Slow-cooker instructions (preferred):

1 Place all the ingredients in a 6-quart slow cooker. Cover and cook on low for 48 hours.

2 Strain broth into jars, discarding bones and other items. Refrigerate, then skim the fat off the top. Reserve the fat for Easy Roasted Potatoes (p. 148).

Stovetop instructions:

1 Place all the ingredients in a large stockpot with a lid. Cover and bring to a boil. Reduce heat and simmer 2 to 8 hours. (The longer it cooks, the richer and more flavorful it will be.)

2 Follow Step 2 of slow-cooker instructions.

Instant Pot instructions:

1 Place all the ingredients in a 6-quart Instant Pot. Secure the lid. Cook on high pressure for 2 hours. Use natural pressure release.

2 Follow Step 2 of slow-cooker instructions.

COOK'S NOTE: *I store chicken bones in a zip-top gallon bag in the freezer, along with any green onion or leek tops. I make broth when the bag is full. If using a smaller amount of bones or a smaller slow cooker or Instant Pot, reduce the water. For example, if your bones fill the slow cooker halfway, add water to just cover them. If making Roasted Chicken with Veggie Gravy (p. 134), toss the giblets into the freezer bag; they add rich nutrition and flavor to your broth. (Make sure the liver is cooked, because it can make the broth bitter if added raw.) To freeze broth: Leave at least 1 inch of room at the top of freezer-safe jars, as it will expand.*

PER 1-CUP SERVING: 1g protein, 0g carbohydrates, 1g fat, 0g saturated fat, 3mg sodium, 10mg potassium, 0g fiber

Perfect Chicken Soup

I first tasted this homemade soup at my friend Carole's house in the Berkshires. She made it with a local heritage chicken, organic vegetables, and spring water. I had no idea chicken soup could taste so amazing. Here's my easy version.

Makes 12 servings

Prep time: 10 minutes
Cooking time: 30 minutes
Passive time: N/A

Budget friendly: Very

8 cups (2L) Low-Sodium Chicken Broth (p. 136)

5 sprigs fresh thyme, tied with kitchen string

3 bay leaves

3 carrots, thickly sliced

3 medium potatoes, diced large

5 stalks celery, thickly sliced

1–2 cups (140–280g) cooked, diced chicken breast, from Roasted Chicken with Veggie Gravy (p. 134)

1 bundle fresh Italian parsley, finely chopped

1 Bring the chicken broth to just under a boil in a large heavy soup pot.

2 Add the thyme and simmer for 10 minutes.

3 Add the bay leaves and vegetables and cook until fork tender, about 10 minutes.

4 Stir in the chicken, and cook for 3 minutes, until hot. Discard the bay leaves and thyme bundle.

5 Ladle soup into bowls and stir about 2 tablespoons of the chopped parsley into each serving. (Add the remaining parsley to the soup before storing in the fridge.)

COOK'S NOTE: *If you don't have homemade chicken broth, use store-bought vegetable or chicken broth. Do not use water. Trust me.*

PER SERVING: 7g protein, 10g carbohydrates, 0g fat, 0g saturated fat, 109mg sodium, 393mg potassium, 2g fiber

Thai-Style Chicken Soup

A delightful chicken soup that is quick to make and loosely based on Thailand's beloved soup, tom yum. I used to order this from restaurants whenever I had a cold or the flu, but had to give it up because of the high sodium content. Now I make it at home, saving a trip while enjoying the vibrant flavors!

Makes 12 servings

Prep time:	10 minutes
Cooking time:	30 minutes
Passive time:	N/A

Budget friendly: Very

8 cups (2L) Low-Sodium Chicken Broth (p. 136)

1 Southeast Asian lime leaf

2–3 stalks lemongrass, pounded lightly to release flavor

6 green onions, thinly sliced on the diagonal

1 shallot, minced (about ¼ cup minced)

1 (8-ounce [225g]) package thin rice noodles (vermicelli)

8 ounces (225g) mushrooms, sliced

1 bunch baby bok choy, thinly sliced (about 2 cups sliced)

1–2 cups (140–280g) cooked, diced chicken breast, from Roasted Chicken with Veggie Gravy (p. 134)

Hot Sauce (p. 196), to taste

Cilantro for garnish (optional)

1 Bring the chicken broth just barely to a boil in a large heavy soup pot.

2 Add the lime leaf, lemongrass, green onions, and shallot and simmer for 10 minutes.

3 Add the noodles and vegetables and cook 10 minutes.

4 Stir in the chicken and cook for 3 minutes, until hot. Discard the lime leaf and lemongrass.

5 Ladle the soup into bowls and season with Hot Sauce. Garnish with minced cilantro if desired.

COOK'S NOTE: *Southeast Asian lime leaves and lemongrass stalks are available at Asian markets. To prepare lemongrass, peel off the outer hard leaves, then finely slice just the soft end near the bulb, discarding the rest. Thin rice noodles are available at most large grocery stores in the Asian section. Choose noodles with just rice as an ingredient. You can use Chile Pepper Sauce (p. 267, The Migraine Relief Plan) in place of the Hot Sauce in this recipe.*

PER SERVING (sodium will be lower with home-cooked chicken):
6g protein, 20g carbohydrates, 1g fat, 1g saturated fat, 180mg sodium, 132mg potassium, 1g fiber

"Expressive writing, if we do it regularly, gives us a visceral experience that things can change—this idea that there are things beyond what we know, and more than one answer. And that is resilience. There's nothing less resilient than feeling stuck."

JEANNINE OUELLETTE, AUTHOR OF *THE PART THAT BURNS*

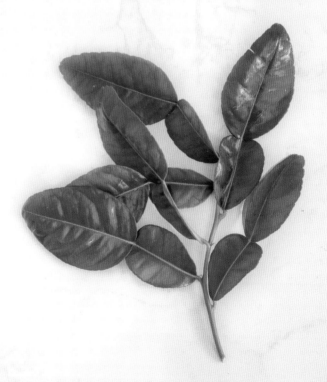

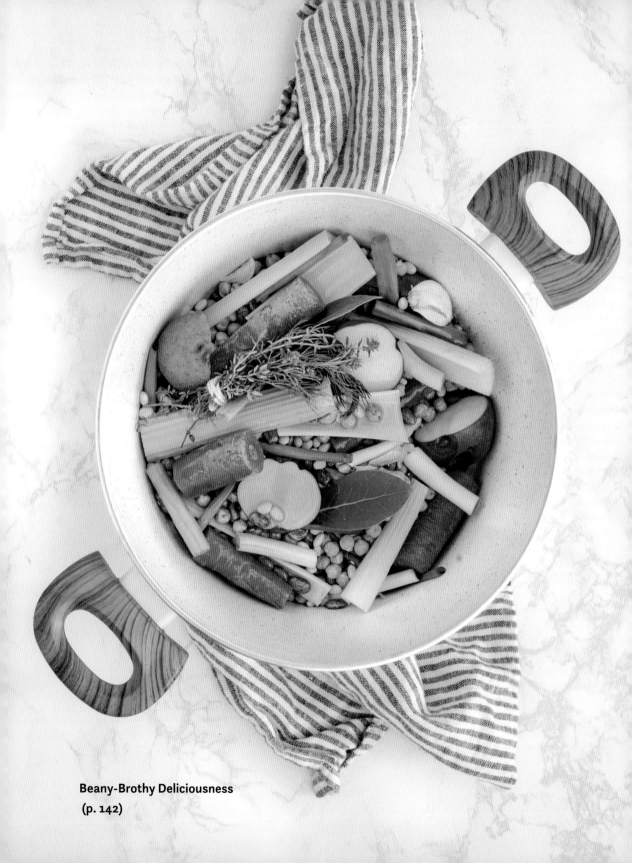

Beany-Brothy Deliciousness
(p. 142)

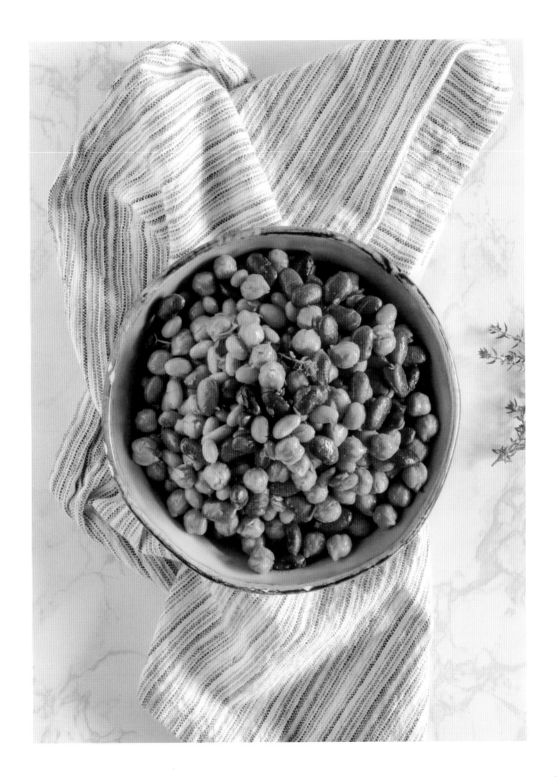

Beany-Brothy Deliciousness

Follow my foolproof method for cooking any type of dried beans and you'll never buy canned again. These perfectly cooked beans are suitable for any number of dishes; as a bonus, they also create a low-sodium vegetable broth and a lovely pureed vegetable soup.

Makes 16 servings

Prep time: 15 minutes
Cooking time: 30 minutes–2 hours
Passive time: 8–12 hours for soaking

Budget friendly: Very

2 cups (450g) dried beans, picked over, rinsed, soaked overnight in filtered water

1 handful fennel fronds

6 fresh thyme sprigs

3 carrots, cut in half

4 stalks celery, whole or cut in half

6 green onions, roots and tips removed

2 cloves garlic, smashed and peeled

2 red or gold potatoes, halved (optional)

2 bay leaves

6 tablespoons (90mL) extra-virgin olive oil

8 cups (2L) filtered water

Stovetop instructions:

1 Drain and rinse the soaked beans before adding to a large cooking pot.

2 Tie the washed fennel fronds and thyme sprigs in a bundle with kitchen twine. Add it to the pot along with all remaining ingredients. Cover.

3 Bring to a boil, then reduce the heat until it's just barely bubbling. Check the beans after 30 minutes. They should be tender but not falling apart. Cook time depends on the size and variety of the beans, anywhere from about 30 minutes to 2 hours.

4 Once the beans are done, discard the herb bundle and bay leaves. Remove the vegetables and set aside for Puréed Vegetable Soup, below.

5 Use a strainer to separate the broth from the beans, making sure to reserve the broth for future use cooking grains or soup.

Instant Pot instructions:

1 Combine all the ingredients. Secure the lid. Select Bean/Chili setting (or use the timing suggested in the manufacturer's recipe booklet for the type of beans you are cooking).

2 Use quick release, covering the valve with a kitchen towel. Continue with Step 4 above.

Puréed Vegetable Soup:

1 Place large chunks of the cooked veggies in a blender with enough broth to make a puréed soup.

PER SERVING (entire recipe made with chickpeas divided by 16):
5g protein, 20g carbohydrates, 6g fat, 1g saturated fat, 42mg sodium, 473mg potassium, 5g fiber

"I maintain a gratitude practice where I come up with three specific, vivid things in the last 24 hours. They can't be the same thing every day. It has to be something different and vivid. Maybe it's imagining a plate of food that you had and all the colors on it. Three things you are grateful for."

MARGOT ANDERSEN, RESILIENCE COACH AND NATIONAL HEADACHE FOUNDATION BOARD MEMBER

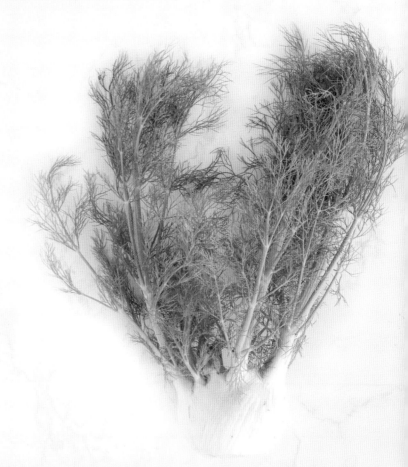

COOK'S NOTE: *Freeze in 1-cup containers so you always have cooked beans ready. Don't skip the fennel, thyme, or bay leaves; they impart essential flavor to the beans. If using a fennel bulb for Tuscan White Bean Soup (p. 144), save the washed fronds, freeze, and use when making these beans. Small beans like chana dal might cook on the stovetop in 30 minutes. Expect about an hour for chickpeas and an hour and 15 minutes for kidney beans. Older beans of any size will take longer to cook, so taste every 30 minutes.*

Tuscan White Bean Soup

I love the flavors of this Italian-inspired soup, which reminds me of a wonderful trip I took with my husband to Florence. It's loaded with an array of vegetables and the fresh, bright flavors and aromas of rosemary, oregano, parsley, and fennel.

Makes 12 servings

Prep time: 10 minutes
Cooking time: 25 minutes
Passive time: N/A

Budget friendly: Very

8 cups (2L) Low-Sodium Chicken Broth (p. 136) or Low-Sodium Vegetable Broth (p. 204)

1 sprig fresh rosemary

3–4 sprigs fresh oregano

1 bulb fennel, diced

1 large zucchini, diced

1 pound (450g) kale, roughly chopped (tough stems removed)

2 cups cooked cannellini beans (see Beany-Brothy Deliciousness, p. 142) or 1 (15.5-ounce [425g]) can low-sodium cannellini beans, rinsed and drained

1 cup (50g) minced Italian parsley (optional)

1 Bring the broth to barely a boil in a large heavy soup pot.

2 Add the rosemary and oregano. Simmer for 10 minutes, adjusting the heat if needed to keep it under a boil.

3 Add the vegetables and beans and cook 10 minutes. Discard the rosemary and oregano stems.

4 Ladle the soup into bowls. Garnish with the parsley, if using.

COOK'S NOTE: *Use Tuscan kale, also called dinosaur or Lacinato kale, for the most authentic flavor. Small packages of herbs are available at most large grocery stores in the produce section. Freeze extra rosemary to use on Easy Roasted Potatoes (p. 148), or stuff inside a chicken the next time you roast one. Using my recipe for Beany-Brothy Deliciousness (p. 142) makes this recipe even lower in sodium. Add diced chicken breast from the Roasted Chicken with Veggie Gravy (p. 134) to make the soup even heartier. Stir it in just after the vegetables are cooked in Step 3 and simmer for about 3 minutes, until chicken is hot. Fennel bulbs and zucchini will vary in size, which might impact the number of servings but not the flavor.*

PER SERVING (using canned beans):
14g protein, 11g carbohydrates, 1g fat, 0g saturated fat, 113mg sodium, 406mg potassium, 3g fiber

Pasta e Fagioli

Enjoy this satisfying, hearty soup of pasta, beans, and vegetables. If you make it with chickpeas, you're making *pasta e ceci*.

Makes 10 servings

Prep time: 20 minutes
Cooking time: 45 minutes
Passive time: N/A

Budget friendly: Very

3 tablespoons extra-virgin olive oil

2 medium carrots, diced

4 ribs celery, diced

6 green onions, thinly sliced

4 cloves garlic, minced

3 bay leaves

2 teaspoons no-salt-added Italian seasoning

1 teaspoon black pepper

4 cups (.95L) Low-Sodium Vegetable Broth (p. 204) or Low-Sodium Chicken Broth (p. 136)

1 (14.5-ounce [411g]) can no-salt-added diced tomatoes

¼ cup (55g) no-salt-added tomato paste

1 cup (250mL) filtered water

8 ounces (225g) gluten-free penne pasta

1 cup cooked chickpeas or cannellini beans (see Beany-Brothy Deliciousness, p. 142) or 1 (15.5-ounce [425g]) can chickpeas or cannellini beans, rinsed and drained

¼ cup (20g) fresh basil, torn

Fresh chèvre (optional)

Stovetop instructions:

1 Heat the oil over medium heat in a large heavy soup pot until shimmering, swirling to coat. Cook the carrots, celery, green onions, garlic, bay leaves, and spices for 5 to 7 minutes until soft but not brown.

2 Add the broth, tomatoes, tomato paste, and water and bring just to a boil. Reduce the heat, cover, and simmer for 15 minutes.

3 Add the pasta and cook for 8 minutes, stirring frequently and adjusting the heat to keep it just bubbling.

4 Add the beans and cook 3 to 4 minutes more until pasta is al dente and the beans are heated through. Discard the bay leaves.

5 Turn off the heat and stir in the basil.

6 Ladle the soup into bowls. Garnish each bowl with a slice of fresh chèvre if using.

Instant Pot instructions:

1 Follow Step 1 above, using Sauté function on medium heat for 5 minutes. Press Cancel.

2 Add the broth, tomatoes, tomato paste, water, and pasta and stir well. Secure the lid. Set to Pressure Cook (high pressure) for 4 minutes. Press Cancel.

3 Use the quick release method with a kitchen towel over the vent to prevent splattering. Open the lid. Discard the bay leaves.

4 Stir in the beans and basil. If pasta is not completely cooked, press Sauté (low setting) and let the soup simmer, tasting every minute or so until pasta is done.

COOK'S NOTE: *To speed up prep: Pulse the carrots, celery, onions, and garlic in a food processor until roughly chopped. Small packages of fresh herbs are available at most large grocery stores in the produce section. Fresh oregano makes a wonderful garnish.*

PER 1-CUP SERVING (using low-sodium canned beans and broth):
5g protein, 32g carbohydrates, 5g fat, 1g saturated fat, 96mg sodium, 489mg potassium, 5g fiber

Quick Bean Tacos

When I need a fast, hearty dinner, I can have this on the table in less than 30 minutes. You can warm the tortillas in a stack in the microwave, but I prefer to heat a pan and toast them while the filling is cooking. Create a taco bar for your family or a party and let people customize their toppings. It's an easy way to feed a crowd and still follow the Plan.

Makes 12 tacos

Prep time: 20 minutes
Cooking time: 10 minutes
Passive time: N/A

Budget friendly: Very

2 tablespoons extra-virgin olive oil

1 bunch green onions (about 6), thinly sliced

4 cups (350g) thinly sliced red cabbage

2 cups cooked pinto beans (see Beany-Brothy Deliciousness, p. 142) or 1 (15.5-ounce [450g]) can low-sodium pinto beans

1 (7-ounce [198g]) can mild green chiles, fire-roasted if available, rinsed and drained

1 (12-ounce [340g]) jar roasted red bell peppers, drained, pressed dry, thinly sliced

12 medium-size fresh corn tortillas

Optional toppings: queso fresco, a fresh Mexican cheese that's reasonably low in sodium, chèvre, Hot Sauce (p. 196), Chile Pepper Sauce (p. 267, *The Migraine Relief Plan*), and minced cilantro

1 Heat the oil over medium heat in a large nonstick sauté pan until shimmering, swirling to coat. Cook the green onions and red cabbage for 5 minutes until glossy and starting to soften.

2 Put the beans and chiles in a colander set over a bowl or in the sink and press with the back of a spoon to release the excess liquid.

3 Add the drained pinto beans, chiles, and red peppers to the pan and stir until bubbling.

4 Preheat a dry grill pan or cast-iron pan over medium-high heat. Lightly spray tortillas on each side with olive oil and toast until crispy but still flexible, 1 to 2 minutes per side.

5 Use ½ cup of filling per tortilla and serve alongside bowls of optional toppings.

COOK'S NOTE: *If you can't find roasted bell peppers in this size jar, this recipe requires 2 to 3 roasted bell peppers.*

 If avocado and lime are not triggers for you, add diced avocado and a squeeze of lime.

PER TACO (using low-sodium canned beans and excluding optional toppings):
5g protein, 41g carbohydrates, 11g fat, 1g saturated fat, 126mg sodium, 433mg potassium, 9g fiber

"I have never stopped making plans, even though I know that I'm going to have to cancel things. I don't stop. I don't ever think, 'Well, I can't ever go to a concert again' or, 'Well, I can't do this.' I always think I'm going to try and maybe it doesn't work out, but that's the biggest thing—I'm going to try. I'm not going to cancel my life because I have a disease. I want to be a participant in it."

EILEEN BREWER, PRESIDENT OF CLUSTERBUSTERS AND THE FOUNDER OF RETREATMIGRAINE

Easy Roasted Potatoes

Potatoes are so satisfying, so plunky (as my husband says), that I had to include this seemingly basic recipe. The key is to lightly coat the potato pieces in healthy fat, then roast at high heat. You'll find the skin to be delightfully crispy, while the inside is fluffy. If you don't eat them all at once, several recipes that follow will make use of the leftovers.

Makes 8 servings

Prep time:	10 minutes
Cooking time:	30–40 minutes
Passive time:	N/A

Budget friendly: Very

2 tablespoons extra-virgin olive oil or chicken fat (p. 136)

2 pounds (900g) organic gold or red new potatoes (approximately 8 small potatoes), cut into 2-inch chunks

1 teaspoon freshly ground black pepper

⅛ teaspoon sea salt (optional)

1 Preheat the oven to 450°F (230°C).

2 On a large, rimmed baking sheet, toss the potatoes with the oil or fat and sprinkle with the pepper and salt (if using). Shake to evenly distribute potatoes across the pan.

3 Roast for 20 minutes, then use a spatula to flip the potatoes.

4 Roast up to 20 minutes more, checking every 10 minutes until the potatoes are crispy and brown on the outside and tender when pierced with a fork.

COOK'S NOTE: *If you don't have a kitchen scale, weigh potatoes at the store. Restaurant supply aisles at large grocery stores or big box stores sell aluminum half sheet pans. These are ideal for roasting pans of vegetables and clean up easily. If you make chicken broth, save the skimmed-off layer of fat to use in this recipe. Try Greek Spice Blend (p. 200) on the potatoes.*

SERVING SUGGESTIONS: Serve with Roasted Chicken with Veggie Gravy (p. 134), Grilled Salmon, Two Glazes (p. 65), Veggie Burgers (p. 71), Beef Barbacoa (p. 102), Lazy Chicken (p. 90), Sheet Pan Chicken Thighs (p. 89), Meatloaf (p. 230, *The Migraine Relief Plan*), Peachy Pulled Pork (p. 234, *The Migraine Relief Plan*), or Chicken or Beef with Pomegranate Marinade (p. 270, *The Migraine Relief Plan*).

PER SERVING (using olive oil and salt): 2g protein, 20g carbohydrates, 4g fat, 1g saturated fat, 37mg sodium, 472mg potassium, 2g fiber

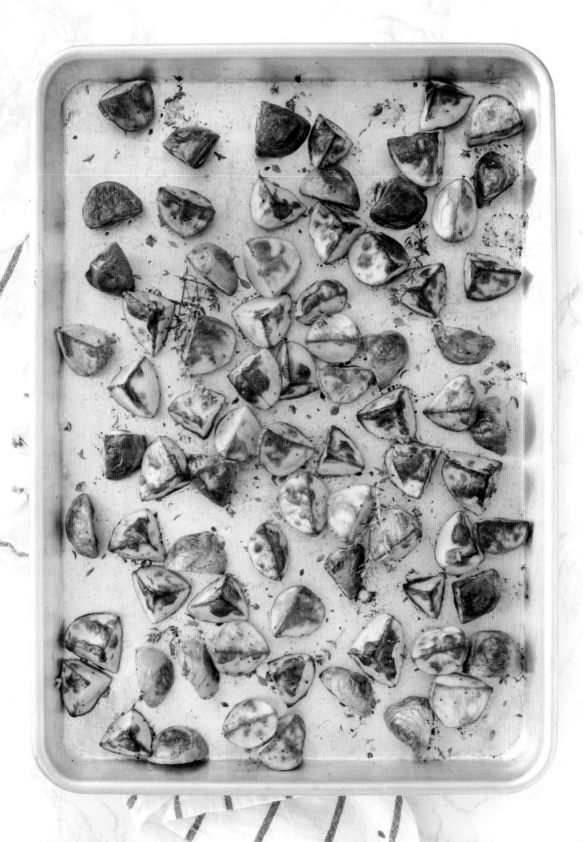

Cauliflower-Chickpea Curry

This recipe is inspired by *aloo gobi*, a turmeric-and-ginger-based Indian dish loaded with potatoes and cauliflower. I've added chickpeas to make this a one-dish meal.

Makes 6 servings

Prep time: 15 minutes
Cooking time: 20–25 minutes
Passive time: N/A

Budget friendly: Very

1 tablespoon extra-virgin coconut or olive oil

3 green onions (40g), thinly sliced

1 tablespoon mild or medium curry powder (can add more in Step 5 if needed)

1 (12-ounce [340g]) package cauliflower florets, separated

1 cup (130g) Easy Roasted Potatoes (p. 148)

2 cups cooked chickpeas (see Beany-Brothy Deliciousness, p. 142) or 1 (15.5-ounce [439g]) can no-salt-added chickpeas, drained

1 (13.5-ounce [400mL]) can coconut milk

½ cup (40g) minced cilantro (optional)

1 Heat the oil in a large pot or Dutch oven over medium heat until shimmering.

2 Sauté the green onions and curry powder for 5 minutes.

3 Add the cauliflower and sauté 3 minutes.

4 Add the potatoes, chickpeas, and coconut milk. Stir well. Bring to a simmer and cook for 10 minutes or until florets are fork tender.

5 Turn off heat and stir in the cilantro if using. Serve as is or over plain basmati rice.

COOK'S NOTE: *You may find canned chickpeas in other sizes, and it's fine to use the entire can (up to 20 ounces [567g]). If you can't find no-salt-added chickpeas, just rinse them well. See the Shopping Guide on page 17 for more information on curry powder. Use half a head of cauliflower if you don't want to use pre-packaged. To make basmati rice: Rinse and drain 1 cup rice 3 times. Add 2 cups filtered water to rice in a medium saucepan. Cover, bring just to a boil, then reduce heat to simmer for 12 minutes. Turn off heat and leave covered for 5 minutes. Fluff with a fork. If you start the rice first, it will be done at the same time as the curry.*

PER 1-CUP SERVING (using coconut oil, no-salt-added canned beans, and roasted potatoes made with salt):
7g protein, 27g carbohydrates, 16g fat, 12g saturated fat, 209mg sodium, 536mg potassium, 3g fiber

"I feel like movement is medicine. It could be yoga, dance, hiking, riding your bike—it doesn't matter what it is, but moving your body to get that energy out. Surrounding yourself with things that support you. I believe that our environment has a great impact. Creating an environment that feels beautiful, nurturing, and honoring to you is extraordinary."

CYNTHIA JAMES, BESTSELLING AUTHOR, INTERNATIONAL SPEAKER AND COACH, HOST OF *WOMEN AWAKENING* PODCAST

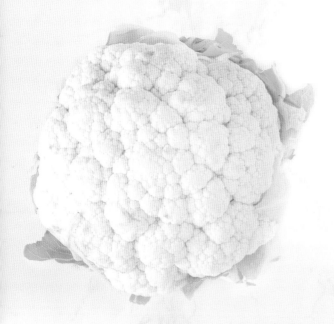

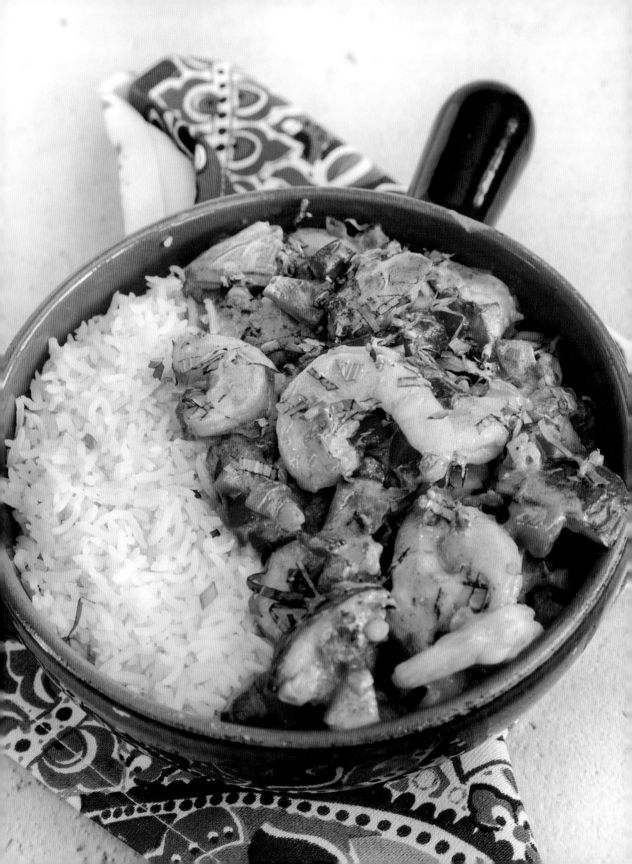

Thai-Style Shrimp Curry

Lovers of Thai food will enjoy this quick shrimp curry, utilizing my Thai red curry paste or store-bought paste, frozen shrimp, and fresh vegetables. If you can, add the fresh basil leaves—they really make it pop!

Makes 5 servings

Prep time: 10 minutes
Cooking time: 23–30 minutes
Passive time: N/A

Budget friendly: Moderate

1 tablespoon extra-virgin coconut or olive oil

2 carrots (1 cup [120g]), diced

1 red bell pepper, diced

1 tablespoon Thai Red Curry Paste (p. 198)

3 green onions (40g), thinly sliced

1 cup (130g) Easy Roasted Potatoes (p. 148)

1 (13.5-ounce [400mL]) can coconut milk

1 pound (450g) wild-caught shrimp, peeled and de-veined, thawed if possible

¼ cup (20g) fresh basil, thinly sliced

1 Heat the oil in a large pot or Dutch oven over medium heat until shimmering.

2 Add the carrots, bell pepper, and curry paste and cook, stirring occasionally, for 10 minutes or until the red bell peppers are golden and softened.

3 Add the green onions and potatoes and sauté 3 minutes.

4 Add the coconut milk. Stir well. Bring to a low boil, then lower the heat and simmer 10 minutes until carrots are just cooked through.

5 Add the shrimp. If using frozen, raise heat to boiling as you add them, and cook until done, up to 10 minutes. If the shrimp are thawed, keep the pan at a simmer and cook for 3 minutes. Shrimp will curl up tightly and feel firm when cooked through.

6 Turn off the heat and stir in the basil if using. Serve as is or over plain basmati rice (see Cook's Note on page 150).

COOK'S NOTE: *Thai red curry paste is usually Plan-friendly except for the high level of sodium. That's why I've included a recipe for making your own (p. 198). If you do, you can freeze it in 1-tablespoon servings (silicone ice cube trays are ideal for this) and pop one out whenever you need it.*

PER 1¼-CUP SERVING (using coconut oil, roasted potatoes with salt, and Thai Kitchen red curry paste):
15g protein, 14g carbohydrates, 19g fat, 15g saturated fat, 333mg sodium, 363mg potassium, 2g fiber

Potato Cakes

Being German, I've never met a potato cake I didn't love. This one is no different. Unlike German potato pancakes, which start with grated raw potato and onion, these begin with my Easy Roasted Potatoes. I use leeks, which are Plan-friendly, instead of onion, and a small amount of brown rice flour to bind them with the eggs. Using a nonstick sauté pan with a small amount of oil produces golden-brown cakes.

Makes 8 cakes

Prep time: 5 minutes
Cooking time: 18–24 minutes
Passive time: N/A

Budget friendly: Very

1 tablespoon extra-virgin coconut or olive oil

1 cup cleaned, thinly sliced leeks (90g)

1 cup (130g) Easy Roasted Potatoes (p. 148), cooled

2 eggs, lightly beaten

2 tablespoons brown-rice flour

1 teaspoon sodium-free baking powder

½ teaspoon freshly ground black pepper

⅛ teaspoon sea salt (optional)

1 Heat the oil in a large nonstick sauté pan over medium heat until shimmering.

2 Sauté the leeks for 5 minutes. Remove from the heat. Do not wipe out pan.

3 Put the sautéed leeks in a food processor fitted with the S-blade and add the potatoes. Pulse in brief pulses 15 times. Mixture should be well broken up but not pureed.

4 Put the potato mixture in a large bowl with the remaining ingredients. Stir just until it comes together.

5 Return the pan to the heat. Scoop even portions of the potato mixture into the pan, smoothing down slightly. Cakes should be 2 inches (5cm) in diameter.

6 Cook 6 to 8 minutes per side, until golden brown and firm. Add additional oil if cakes are sticking. Serve with mayonnaise, unsweetened applesauce, or Hot Sauce (p. 196).

COOK'S NOTE: *I use a #24 (1.5 fl. oz/44 mL) disher scoop, which is equivalent to a standard ¼ cup or a small ice cream scoop. Other possible toppings from* The Migraine Relief Plan: *Chile Pepper Sauce (p. 267), Cilantro Mayonnaise (p. 268), Ranch Dressing (p. 272), or Smoky Mustard Sauce (p. 273).*

PER 2-INCH CAKE (using olive oil, roasted potatoes made with salt, and optional salt):
2g protein, 6g carbohydrates, 3g fat, 1g saturated fat, 85mg sodium, 115mg potassium, 1g fiber

"I developed a self-care practice that I call CARE. The letters stand for Check-in: really noticing what's happening in the mind and body in the present moment by asking the question, 'What's here now?' Acknowledgment (or acceptance): register what's happening in the present moment and don't push it away. Responding: with kindness and self-compassion is really important for me, and asking the question, 'What's needed now?' Embodiment: as you continue to practice CARE, it becomes second nature and you embody this practice."

SHIRLEY KESSEL, EXECUTIVE DIRECTOR OF MILES FOR MIGRAINE

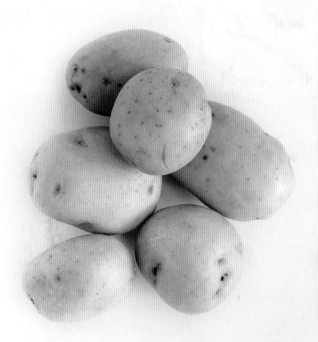

Tex-Mex Skillet Dinner

If you grew up on Hamburger Helper like I did, this dish hits some of those notes without additives like whey, wheat flour, and cornstarch. It's not true Tex-Mex food, but echoes the flavors of a tasty fajita dinner.

Makes 5 servings

Prep time: 5 minutes
Cooking time: 20–25 minutes
Passive time: N/A

Budget friendly: Moderate

1 pound (450 g) 90% lean grass-fed ground beef

1 tablespoon Taco Seasoning (p. 202), or more to taste

6 green onions (80g), thinly sliced

3 ribs celery, thinly sliced

1 red bell pepper, medium diced

1 cup (130g) Easy Roasted Potatoes (p. 148), medium diced

½ cup (40g) cilantro (optional)

1 Cook the beef with the Taco Seasoning in a large nonstick pot or stainless-steel Dutch oven over medium heat until browned, breaking up the meat with a spoon. After 10 minutes, use paper towels to blot any excess oil.

2 Add the green onions, celery, and peppers and cook 6 to 8 minutes until golden and softened.

3 Add the potatoes and cook until heated through.

4 Turn off the heat. Stir in the cilantro (if using).

COOK'S NOTE: *If using ground chicken or ground turkey for this dish, start the sauté pan with 1 tablespoon extra-virgin olive oil. Feel free to add a minced jalapeño or cayenne pepper to spice this up.*

PER 1-CUP SERVING (using roasted potatoes made with salt):
19g protein, 11g carbohydrates, 10g fat, 14g saturated fat, 172mg sodium, 381mg potassium, 2g fiber

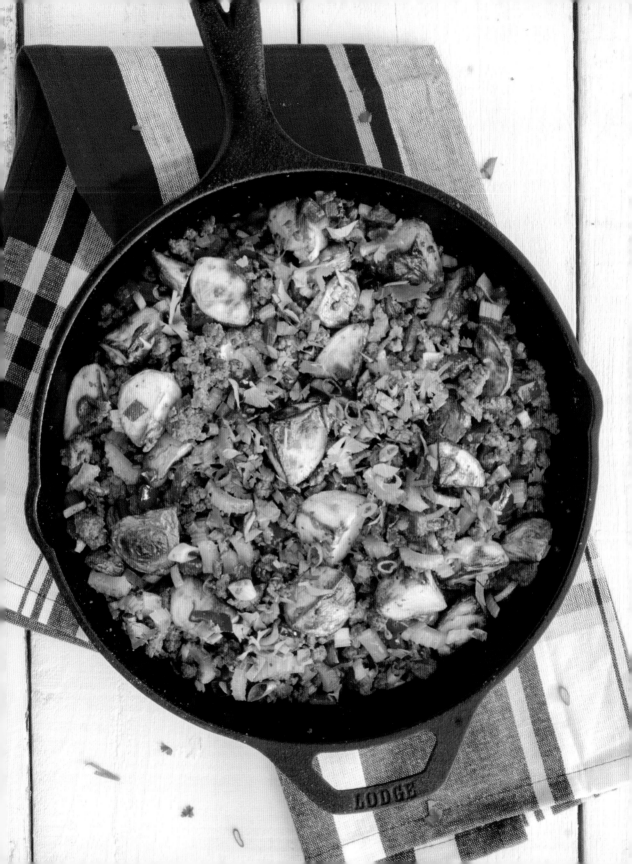

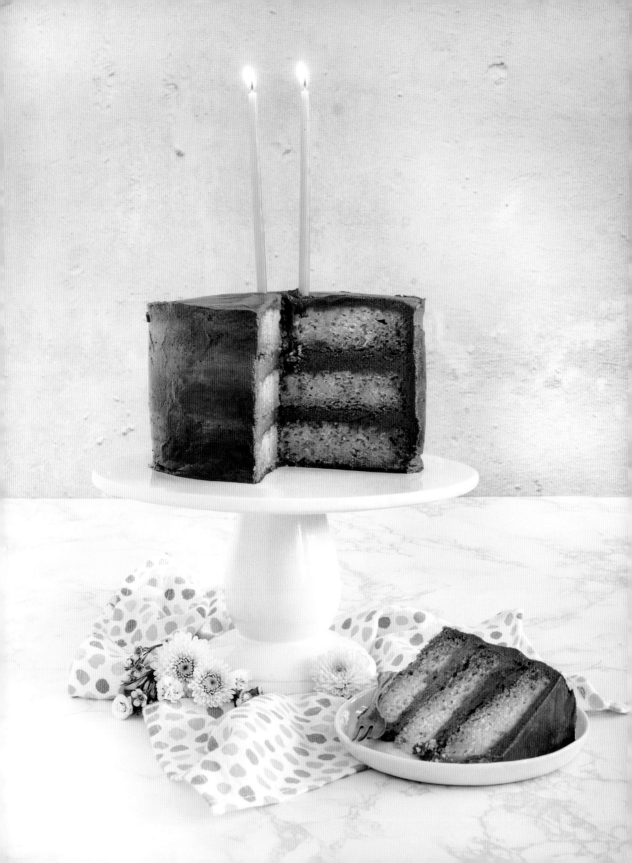

Desserts

I love desserts and wanted to provide a variety for people following my Plan. These range from very simple, like a mug cake cooked in the microwave or "fudge" made in the freezer, to pies and a beautiful cake for special occasions. And with frozen desserts, a pudding, and fruity gelatin, kids will love them too.

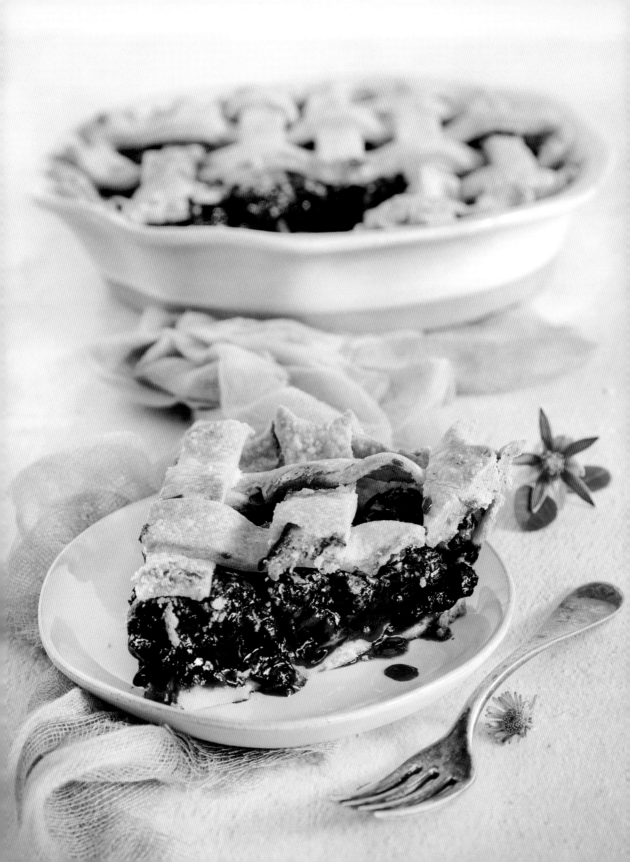

Blueberry Pie

There's something so summery about blueberry pie, especially when it's made using those fat juicy berries that show up in mid-July. Maybe I love it because it's nearly purple when baked, and that's my favorite color.

Makes 8 servings

Prep time: 20 minutes
Cooking time: 35–40 minutes
Passive time: 30 minutes for cooling

Budget friendly: Moderate

¼ cup (30g) tapioca flour or arrowroot powder

1 teaspoon cinnamon

Stevia to equal 3 teaspoons sugar

½ teaspoon white vinegar

3 cups (1.5 pounds [650g]) blueberries, thawed and well drained if frozen

2 Gluten-Free Pastry Crusts (p. 162)

1 Mix the tapioca, cinnamon, and stevia in a small bowl. Add the vinegar, stirring until well mixed. Pour this mixture over the blueberries in a large bowl, stirring to combine completely. Set aside while you make the crust.

2 Preheat the oven to 375°F (190°C).

3 Prepare the Gluten-Free Pastry Crusts as instructed on page 162. Place the bottom crust (waxed paper removed) into an 8-inch (20cm) pie pan. Pour in the blueberry filling.

4 Remove the top sheet of waxed paper from the second crust and place it, crust side down, over the blueberry filling. Peel off the second sheet of waxed paper.

5 Pinch the top and bottom crusts firmly together around the edges so they're completely sealed, and trim off any excess. Cut slits in the center to allow steam to escape.

6 Put the pie on a baking sheet to catch potential drips and help crisp the bottom.

7 Bake for 35 to 40 minutes. It's ready when the crust is light golden brown and the filling begins to bubble up. It often boils over in the last 3 or 4 minutes.

8 Place on a wire rack to cool completely. The filling will firm up the longer it sits, and it will get very firm on day three—if the pie lasts that long.

COOK'S NOTE: *Tapioca starch, also called tapioca flour, creates a firmer filling.*

PER SERVING (with crusts made using Bob's Red Mill Gluten Free 1-to-1 Baking Flour):
3g protein, 57g carbohydrates, 6g fat, 5g saturated fat, 26mg sodium, 67mg potassium, 4g fiber

Gluten-Free Pastry Crust

I have been disappointed in so many store-bought gluten-free crusts. Making them from scratch is a challenge; the dough is difficult to roll out, cracks easily, and isn't always flaky. Then I remembered my mother's cream cheese crust recipe. This pastry is a dream to work with and I'm positive it will turn out for you.

Makes 1 crust fitting an 8- or 9-inch pie pan, with dough left over

Prep time: 5 minutes
Cooking time: N/A
Passive time: 5–10 minutes if chilling dough

Budget friendly: Moderate

If doubling this recipe I recommend making each crust separately.

1 cup (148g) gluten-free flour such as Bob's Red Mill Gluten Free 1-to-1 Baking Flour or my Gluten-Free Flour Blend (p. 203), sifted or fluffed, then leveled

4 ounces (115g) cold butter, cut into pieces

3 ounces (85g) cold cream cheese, cut into pieces

1 Put all the ingredients in a food processor and process for about 25 seconds until dough comes together in a ball. (If not using right away, dough can be well-wrapped and frozen for 2 months. Thaw overnight in the refrigerator before using, then proceed to Step 2.)

2 Roll out the dough between two sheets of 12-inch (30cm) square waxed paper to ⅛-inch (4mm) thick. The dough circle should reach the edges of the square. If it's sticking, chill for 5 to 10 minutes.

3 Peel off the top layer of waxed paper. Place the dough into a pie pan, removing the other sheet of waxed paper as you press it into the pan. Trim away excess dough and form a rolled or decorative edge.

COOK'S NOTE: *I have tested this recipe with four commercial one-to-one flour blends as well as my Gluten-Free Flour Blend (p. 203), so I know it will work in any kitchen. Read your gluten-free flour blend label; if it does not include xanthan gum, you'll need to whisk in 1 teaspoon psyllium husk powder as a binder. Make use of extra pastry by decorating the top or making a hand pie. If you refrigerate the dough, set it out on the counter for at least 15 minutes, until pliable, before rolling out. You can use this crust to make empanadas, any of the pies in this book, and Quiche (p. 285, The Migraine Relief Plan). If you'd like to pre-roll and freeze the dough in a pie tin, wrap it very well before freezing, then thaw on the counter before baking. To use the crust with a no-bake filling, follow the instructions through Step 3. Prick the bottom of the crust all over with a fork, then place a square of parchment paper inside the shell and fill with dried beans or pie weights. Bake at 425°F (220°C) for 15 minutes, remove the parchment and the weights, then bake another 5 to 7 minutes until golden across the bottom. Cool completely.*

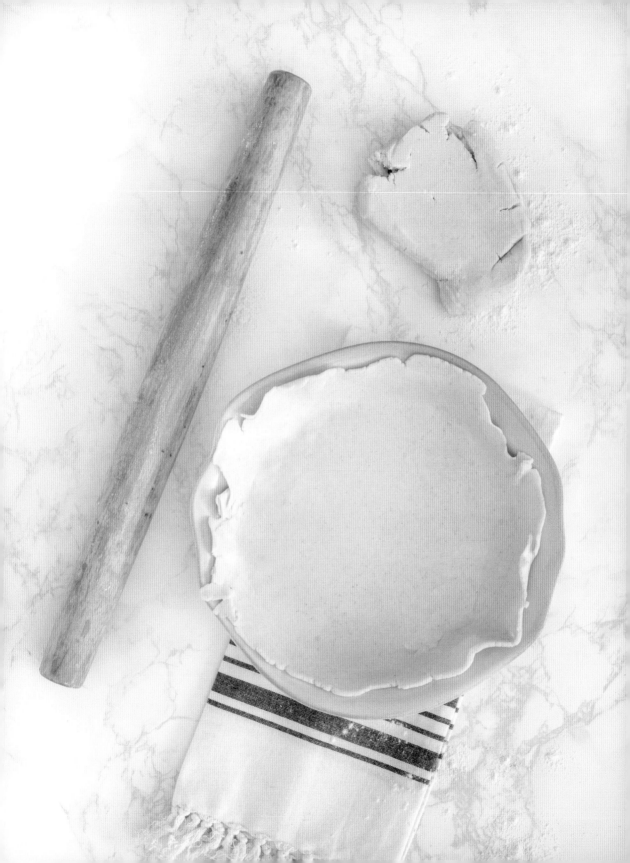

Cherry Pie

My favorite pie memory is the holiday meal where my entire family sat down to dig into Mom's sour-cherry pie. Our mouths puckered into identical Os of surprise, as Mom had forgotten to put in the sugar. No need to worry about that here, as we start with sweet cherries.

Makes 8 servings

Prep time: 15 minutes
Cooking time: 35–50 minutes
Passive time: 15–30 minutes

Budget friendly: Moderate, depending on price of fruit

2 tablespoons tapioca flour or arrowroot powder

½ teaspoon ground nutmeg

½ teaspoon cinnamon

Stevia to equal 4 teaspoons sugar

½ teaspoon white vinegar

3 cups (1.5 pounds [650g]) fresh or frozen sweet cherries, pitted, thawed and drained well

2 Gluten-Free Pastry Crusts (p. 162)

1 Mix the tapioca, nutmeg, cinnamon, and stevia in a small bowl then add the vinegar, stirring until well mixed. Pour this mixture over the cherries in a large bowl, stirring to combine completely.

2 Preheat the oven to 375°F (190°C).

3 Prepare the Gluten-Free Pastry Crusts as instructed on page 162. Place the bottom crust (waxed paper removed) into an 8-inch (20cm) pie pan. Pour in the cherry filling.

4 Remove the top sheet of waxed paper from the second crust and place it, crust side down, over the filling. Peel off the second sheet of waxed paper.

5 Pinch the top and bottom crust together firmly around the edges so they're completely sealed, and trim off any excess dough. Cut slits in the center to allow steam to escape.

6 Put the pie on a baking sheet to catch potential drips and help crisp the bottom.

7 Bake for 35 minutes. If it's light golden brown and you're starting to see the filling bubble up, pull it out. It often boils over in the last 3 or 4 minutes. If not, bake for up to 50 minutes.

8 Place on a wire rack to cool completely. The filling will firm up the longer it sits, and will get very firm on day three—if the pie lasts that long.

COOK'S NOTE: *Tapioca starch, also called tapioca flour, creates a firmer filling. Do not use canned sour cherries for this recipe; the stevia is not sweet enough. Pit fresh cherries using a chopstick if you do not have a cherry pitter.*

PER SERVING (with Bob's Red Mill Gluten Free 1-to-1 Baking Flour):
4g protein, 58g carbohydrates, 19g fat, 15g saturated fat, 25mg sodium, 189mg potassium, 3g fiber

Peach Crumble Pie

Every summer when stone fruit come into season, I'll make one perfect peach pie. I love how the crumble topping adds texture and enhances the sweet blush of the peaches.

Makes 8 servings

Prep time: 15 minutes
Cooking time: 35–40 minutes
Passive time: 30 minutes

Budget friendly: Moderate

¼ cup (30g) plus 1 tablespoon tapioca flour or arrowroot powder, divided

1½ teaspoons cinnamon, divided

¼ teaspoon ground nutmeg

¼ teaspoon ground ginger

Stevia to equal 4 teaspoons sugar (can omit if peaches are very sweet)

¼ teaspoon white vinegar

2 pounds (900g) fresh or frozen peaches, about 8 medium, peeled and sliced, thawed if frozen

¼ cup (35g) raw sunflower seeds

¼ cup (30g) coconut flour

¼ cup (40g) coconut sugar

4 tablespoons butter or coconut oil, chilled

1 Gluten-Free Pastry Crust (p. 162), placed in a pie pan with a rolled-edge crust

1 Preheat the oven to 375°F (190°C).

2 Whisk ¼ cup of the tapioca flour, ½ teaspoon of the cinnamon, the nutmeg, the ginger, the stevia, and the vinegar in a large bowl, then toss with the peaches until combined. Set aside.

3 Put the sunflower seeds, coconut flour, coconut sugar, butter, and the remaining 1 tablespoon tapioca flour in a food processor and pulse 8 to 10 times until the mixture looks like small peas or fine gravel. Set aside.

4 Pour the peach filling into the crust. Spread the crumble mixture evenly over the filling with your fingers.

5 Put the pie on a baking sheet to catch potential drips and help crisp the bottom.

6 Bake pie for 35 to 40 minutes, checking after 20 minutes. If the crumble is getting too brown, cover lightly with foil. Begin checking every 10 minutes until filling is bubbly and crumble is golden brown.

7 Place the pie on a wire rack to cool completely. The filling will firm up the longer it sits, and will get very firm on day three—if the pie lasts that long.

COOK'S NOTE: *To peel fresh peaches, cut an × on the bottom of each peach and drop into boiling water for 2 to 3 minutes. Allow to cool, then rub off the skins and slice. If using frozen peaches, discard any pieces that are very brown or bruised. Tapioca starch, also called tapioca flour, creates a firmer filling. One tester successfully substituted organic brown sugar for the coconut sugar.*

PER SERVING (with Bob's Red Mill Gluten Free 1-to-1 Baking Flour and coconut oil):
4g protein, 45g carbohydrates, 18g fat, 8g saturated fat, 44mg sodium, 239mg potassium, 4g fiber

Pumpkin Pie

Thanksgiving is not the same without it. Even if I'm not eating a traditional meal anymore, I have to bake pumpkin pie. My mom made the best, so I adapted her version for the Plan. If needed for you or someone you love, you can make this dairy- and grain-free by omitting the crust.

Makes 8 servings

Prep time:	5 minutes (excluding crust)
Cooking time:	50–60 minutes
Passive time:	30 minutes

Budget friendly: Very

1 Gluten-Free Pastry Crust (p. 162), see Cook's Note

1 (15-ounce [425g]) can pumpkin puree

¾ cup (175 mL) whole, hemp, or coconut milk

¼ cup (40g) coconut sugar

3 eggs

½ teaspoon cinnamon

¼ teaspoon dried ginger

Pinch ground nutmeg

Pinch ground cloves

Stevia equal to 4 teaspoons sugar

1 Preheat oven to 350°F (180°C).

2 Place one Gluten-Free Pastry Crust in your pie pan. If making pie without a crust, grease pie pan.

3 Blend all the remaining ingredients until smooth in a blender or food processor. Pour into the prepared pie pan.

4 Bake 50 to 60 minutes on the center rack of the oven until the center of the pie is set with some cracks, a toothpick comes out clean, and crust (if using) is golden.

5 Cool completely on a wire rack before serving.

COOK'S NOTE: *Add more stevia if you want a sweeter pie, up to the equivalent of 8 teaspoons. Top with Coconut Whipped Cream (p. 254,* The Migraine Relief Plan*).*

PER SERVING (with Gluten-Free Pastry Crust and hemp milk):
4g protein, 26g carbohydrates, 12g fat, 8g saturated fat, 49mg sodium, 26mg potassium, 2g fiber

PER SERVING (without crust, with hemp milk):
3g protein, 11g carbohydrates, 3g fat, 1g saturated fat, 38mg sodium, 26mg potassium, 2g fiber

Apple-Spice Mug Cake

Ever have one of those days when you think, I would love just a little treat? Mug cake recipes were all the rage a few years back on the internet. Stir a few ingredients, microwave, and suddenly you have a single serving of warm cake! You'll love the flavor and texture, and that it only leaves one mug to clean.

Makes 1 serving

Prep time:	7 minutes
Cooking time:	2 minutes
Passive time:	N/A

Budget friendly: Very

1 egg

2 tablespoons whole, hemp, or light coconut milk

1 teaspoon vanilla extract

Stevia to equal 1 teaspoon sugar

¼ cup gluten-free flour such as Bob's Red Mill 1-to-1 Baking Flour or my Gluten-Free Flour Blend (p. 203)

¼ teaspoon Pumpkin Pie Spice (p. 200)

1 medium apple, very finely chopped, unpeeled

1 Add the egg to a microwave-safe mug and beat lightly with a fork. Add the rest of the ingredients in the order listed, mixing with a fork as you add each one.

2 Microwave for 1 minute, then in 15-second increments, checking the cake each time. Total time will depend on the microwave. Cake should puff up and feel firm. Don't overcook or it will dry out. Eat while still warm.

COOK'S NOTE: *Make sure you add the ingredients in the order listed, and stir after each one. Make sure the apple pieces are tiny, so they cook enough.*

"I don't just drink a cup of coffee; I make sure that I savor at least the first sip. I take a moment to look out the window and focus on the shapes of the leaves on the plants. I put on my favorite song and really listen to it, rather than having it as background music. My self-care practice isn't big things that take time or money, like getting a massage or even taking a bubble bath. It's about incorporating activities that nourish me into everyday life."

KERRIE SMYRES, *THE DAILY HEADACHE*

PER SERVING (with light coconut milk):
9g protein, 53g carbohydrates, 6g fat, 3g saturated fat, 86mg sodium, 245mg potassium, 6g fiber

Cheesecake

Yes, you can have cheesecake on the Plan! Enjoy this luscious treat on special occasions. With only 7 grams of carbs, it's suitable for diabetics too.

Makes 12 servings

Prep time: 30 minutes
Cooking time: 60–75 minutes
Passive time: 4+ hours

Budget friendly: Moderate

3½ cups (120g) puffed rice cereal or 1 cup (120g) sunflower seeds

4–6 tablespoons (60–90g) softened butter or extra-virgin coconut oil, divided

15–16 ounces (425–450g) whole-milk ricotta cheese

8 ounces (225g) regular cream cheese

3 eggs

2 tablespoons coconut flour

Stevia to equal 8 teaspoons sugar

1 tablespoon best-quality pure vanilla extract

Fresh berries for garnish

1 Preheat oven to 325°F (165°C).

2 Process the cereal or seeds into fine crumbs in a food processor fitted with the S-blade. Add 2 tablespoons of the butter or oil and pulse to combine. The mixture should hold together when pressed. If not, add more fat 1 tablespoon at a time until it does.

3 Press the mixture evenly into the bottom and halfway up the sides of an oiled 9-inch (20 to 24cm) springform pan. Use a piece of waxed paper to help you press it evenly. Bake 5 to 7 minutes until light golden brown, then set on a cooling rack. Leave the oven on.

4 Add the cheeses, eggs, coconut flour, stevia, and vanilla to the bowl of a food processor or mixer and puree until very smooth, stopping to scrape down the sides as needed.

5 Brush the sides of the pan (above the crust) with the remaining melted butter or coconut oil.

6 Pour the filling into the crust. Let stand for 10 minutes to allow air bubbles to rise to the top. Gently rake the surface with a fork to break any air bubbles.

7 Bake 45 to 60 minutes until the filling is set, the top cracks, and the edges are golden brown.

8 Turn the oven off and let cake sit inside for one hour.

9 Place cheesecake on a wire rack to cool completely, at least 4 hours. Refrigerate until 30 minutes before serving.

10 Run a knife between the cheesecake and the pan before releasing the pan. Garnish slices with fresh berries.

COOK'S NOTE: *In the US, ricotta cheese is sold in both 15- and 16-ounce containers. Either works. Berry Sauce (p. 250,* The Migraine Relief Plan*) makes an excellent topping. Use sunflower seeds for the crust to make this grain-free.*

PER SERVING (with puffed rice cereal, 4 tablespoons coconut oil, 15 ounces whole-milk ricotta):
8g protein, 7g carbohydrates, 15g fat, 7g saturated fat, 136mg sodium, 74mg potassium, 1g fiber

Dutch Apple Cake

This is one of only three family recipes I have that reflect my German-Lutheran heritage. The crust is more biscuit-like than cakey, and pairs well with spicy herbal tea.

Makes 9 servings

Prep time: 30 minutes
Cooking time: 45–50 minutes
Passive time: 10–15 minutes

Budget friendly: Very

2 tablespoons pure maple syrup

1 tablespoon butter or coconut oil, melted

¾ teaspoons cinnamon, divided

1 cup (148g) gluten-free flour such as Bob's Red Mill Gluten Free 1-to-1 Baking Flour or my Gluten-Free Flour Blend (p. 203), sifted and fluffed, then leveled

Stevia to equal 2 teaspoons sugar

2 teaspoons sodium-free baking soda substitute (see Shopping Guide, p. 17), or 1½ teaspoons regular baking soda

¼ teaspoon ground cloves

¼ teaspoon ground nutmeg

¼ cup (45g) butter or coconut oil, chilled

1 egg

¼ cup (60mL) half and half or coconut milk

3 medium baking apples, such as Granny Smith, peeled and cored

1 Preheat the oven to 375°F (190°C). Oil an 8- or 9-inch (20 or 23cm) square baking pan.

2 Make a glaze by mixing the maple syrup, melted butter, and ¼ teaspoon of the cinnamon in a small bowl. Set aside.

3 In a large mixing bowl, whisk together the flour, stevia, baking soda, cloves, nutmeg, and the remaining cinnamon until one color.

4 Cut the chilled butter or coconut oil into the flour mixture with a pastry cutter, fork, or two knives until the fat is evenly mixed through the flour. It should look like crumbly sand with no large lumps.

5 Whisk together the egg and half and half or coconut milk in a small bowl, then add it to the flour bowl and mix with a spatula until incorporated.

6 Cut one apple into chunks and pulse in a food processor fitted with the S-blade until finely chopped. Stir apple into the batter until evenly incorporated. Let the batter rest 10 minutes. Meanwhile, cut the remaining two apples into thin wedges.

7 Spread the batter into the prepared pan in an even layer. Brush a light coating of the glaze on top, then press apples point-side-down into the batter in rows until they touch the bottom of the pan. Use a pastry brush to spread the remaining glaze over the top of the cake, coating all the apples.

8 Bake for 35 minutes or until cake is golden brown in the center and caramelizing on the edges. The center should spring back when pressed with a finger.

9 Let cool on a wire rack. Use a very sharp knife to cut it into 9 squares.

COOK'S NOTE: *Granny Smith or another firm baking apple are perfect for this recipe. This tastes best made with butter or ghee (especially in the glaze). Boiled cider syrup (recipes online) adds an intense layer of flavor and may be substituted for the maple syrup.*

PER SERVING (with coconut oil, coconut milk, and baking soda substitute):
2g protein, 25g carbohydrates, 10g fat, 8g saturated fat, 14mg sodium, 75mg potassium, 2g fiber

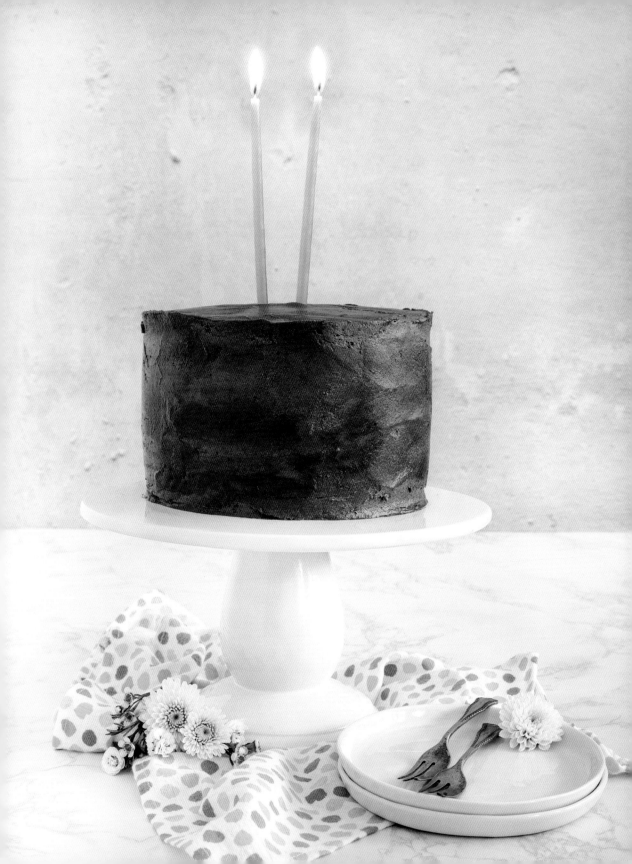

Birthday Cake with Fudgy Frosting

To celebrate the two-year anniversary of the publication of *The Migraine Relief Plan*, I asked the readers in my Facebook group what recipe they wanted. The answer? Birthday cake! Yes, there's a little sugar in this. Because you only celebrate birthdays once in a while.

Makes one 2- or 3-layer cake or 18 cupcakes

Prep time: 30 minutes
Cooking time: 20–40 minutes
Passive time: 30 minutes

Budget friendly: Moderate

2 eggs, separated

2 cups gluten-free flour such as Bob's Red Mill 1-to-1 Baking Flour or my Gluten-Free Flour Blend (p. 203)

2 ½ teaspoons baking powder

½ teaspoon sodium-free baking soda substitute (see Shopping Guide, p. 17)

¾ cup (180mL) agave syrup, honey, or maple syrup

¾ cup (180mL) whole, coconut, hemp, or rice milk

⅓ cup (80mL) grapeseed, sunflower seed, or light olive oil

2 tablespoons vanilla extract

Fudgy Frosting (recipe follows)

1 Preheat the oven to 350°F (180°C).

2 Grease 2 (8-inch) or 3 (6-inch) cake pans and line bottoms with parchment paper circles or line 18 cupcake tins with liners.

3 Beat the egg whites with a handheld or stand mixer until stiff peaks form. Set aside.

4 In a medium bowl, whisk the flour, baking powder, and baking soda until combined.

5 In a mixing bowl (or the bowl of a stand mixer), beat the egg yolks, agave syrup, coconut milk, oil, and vanilla until smooth.

6 Add the flour mixture and beat until no lumps remain. Fold in the egg whites using a spatula, until mixed in completely.

7 Divide the batter evenly between the 2 or 3 cake pans (use a kitchen scale to get the layers the same weight) or scoop into prepared cupcake tins, about ⅔ full.

8 Place on the oven's center rack. Bake 8-inch cakes 35 to 40 minutes and 6-inch cakes 20 to 25 minutes, rotating pans halfway through the baking time. Bake cupcakes 10 minutes, then rotate the pans and bake another 8 to 10 minutes, or until tops spring back and a toothpick comes out clean. Cool cakes for 15 minutes in the pans before removing to a wire rack to finish cooling. Cool cupcakes completely on wire racks before frosting.

COOK'S NOTE: *If you are not following a low-sodium diet, use regular baking soda. If using a gluten-free flour blend that does not contain xanthan gum or psyllium husk powder, add 1½ teaspoons psyllium husk powder in Step 4 of the cake recipe. This cake tastes best the day it's baked. Warm briefly in a microwave on day two. The cake in the photograph was made using three 6-inch cake pans. If you want to pipe rosettes on top, it will require a double batch of frosting.*

Adapted from Golden Vanilla Cake or Cupcakes and Chocolate Buttercream Frosting from Naturally Sweet and Gluten-Free *by Ricki Heller.*

PER CUPCAKE: 6g protein, 51g carbohydrates, 12g fat, 4g saturated fat, 158mg sodium, 11mg potassium, 3g fiber

Fudgy Frosting

1 cup (170g) organic coconut sugar

1 cup (245g) sweet potato puree (canned or home-baked)

40 drops organic stevia drops, vanilla flavor preferred, or powdered stevia to equal 8 teaspoons sugar

4 teaspoons vanilla extract

½ cup (40g) unsweetened carob powder

½ cup (75g) unsweetened carob chips

½ cup (128g) tahini or no-salt-added sunflower seed butter

¼ cup (60mL) coconut oil

1 Place the coconut sugar in a blender and blend on high for 1 minute to make a fine powder.

2 Transfer the powdered coconut sugar to a food processor fitted with the S-blade and add the sweet potato and stevia. Process until smooth.

3 Place the remaining ingredients (vanilla extract through coconut oil) in a heavy-bottomed saucepan and stir over medium-low heat until melted and smooth. Scrape into the food processor with the sweet potato mixture. Blend until very smooth.

4 For thick fudgy frosting, immediately spread on cupcakes. For pipeable buttercream-style frosting, refrigerate until cold then beat until very fluffy. Use a large piping tip to create frosting swirls.

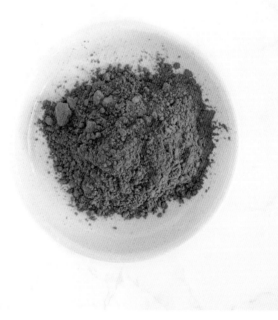

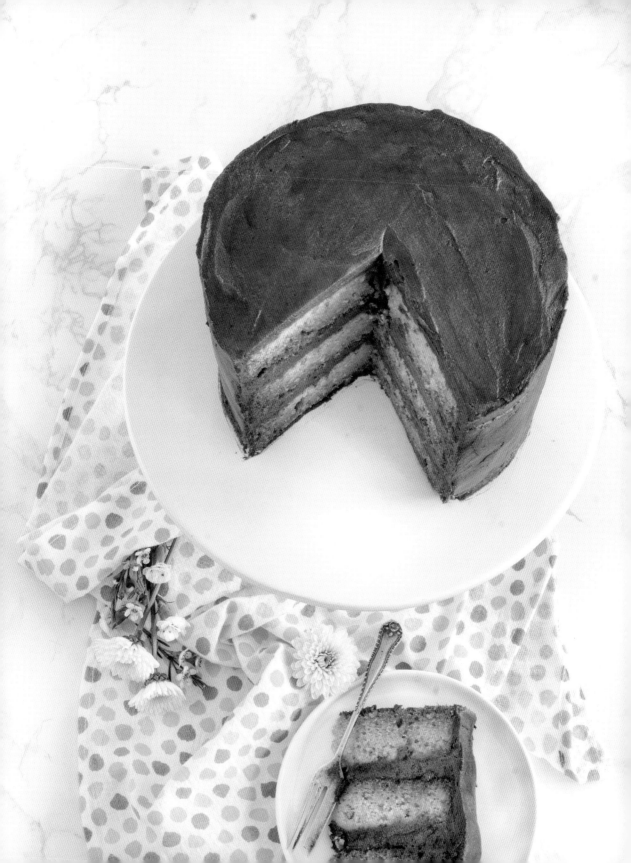

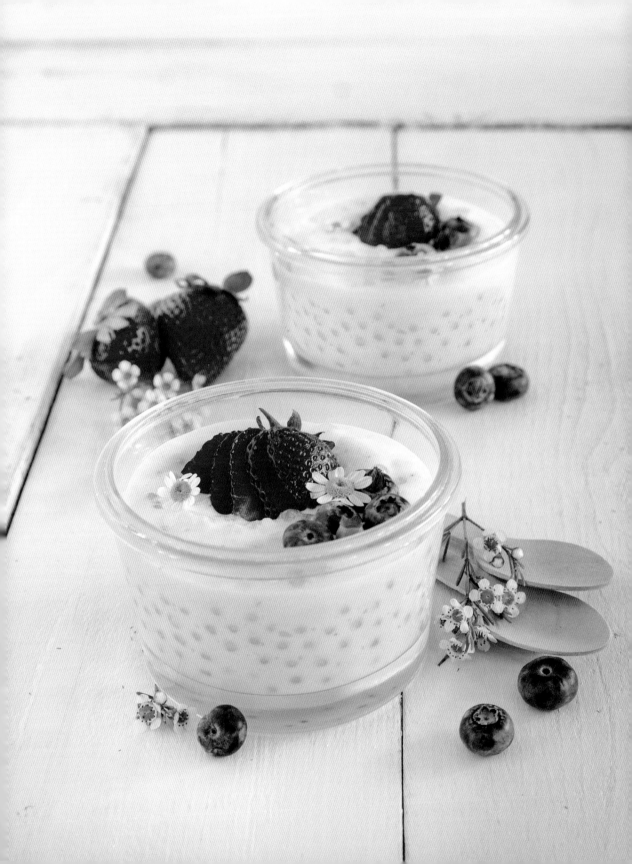

Tapioca Pudding

We had pudding often in my house growing up, usually from a boxed mix. But my mom always made tapioca pudding from scratch, and it's one of my favorite dessert memories from childhood. I still love the squishy pearls floating in the cloudlike pudding.

Makes 6 servings

Prep time: 5 minutes
Cooking time: 25–30 minutes
Passive time: 45+ minutes

Budget friendly: Very

⅓ cup (55g) small pearl tapioca

¾ cup (180mL) filtered water

2 eggs, separated

2¼ cups (560mL) whole, rice, coconut, or hemp milk

Stevia to equal 4 teaspoons sugar

1 tablespoon vanilla extract

½ cup (25g) unsweetened finely shredded coconut flakes (optional)

¼ teaspoon ground nutmeg

1 Combine the tapioca and water in a saucepan and let soak for 30 minutes.

2 Put the egg yolks in a small bowl and beat them lightly with a fork.

3 Whisk the milk and egg yolks into the tapioca-water mixture in the saucepan and cook uncovered over medium-high heat just until boiling.

4 Reduce the heat to a simmer and cook over low heat for 10 minutes, stirring often, until tapioca has doubled in size and is translucent and pudding has noticeably thickened.

5 Place the egg whites in a mixing bowl (or the bowl of a stand mixer), add the stevia, and beat on high speed until soft peaks form.

6 Add about 1 cup of the hot tapioca mixture, a little at a time, into the egg whites with a spatula, then fold the mixture back into the saucepan. (This keeps the egg whites from cooking.)

7 Stir over low heat for 3 minutes.

8 Remove from the heat and cool 15 minutes, then stir in the vanilla, coconut (if using), and nutmeg.

9 Pour into a serving bowl and refrigerate until set, at least 30 minutes. Once cool, cover the bowl if not serving right away.

COOK'S NOTE: *You may substitute large pearl tapioca but not granulated tapioca or tapioca flour for this recipe. If using liquid stevia, start with 15 drops and see if it is sweet enough for your taste. Freshly grated nutmeg adds amazing flavor.*

PER SERVING (with hemp milk and coconut flakes):
3g protein, 9g carbohydrates, 7g fat, 3g saturated fat, 71mg sodium, 27mg potassium, 1g fiber

Strawberry Sorbet

A delightful frozen treat, which can also be made with frozen strawberries. If using fresh, be sure to choose organic berries at the peak of sweetness. This is a hit with kids.

Makes 6 servings

Prep time: 5 minutes
Cooking time: N/A
Passive time: 30–60 minutes (for chilling and churning)

Budget friendly: Very

1 pound (450g) organic strawberries, hulled, thawed if frozen

¾ cup (180mL) coconut cream or heavy cream

2 tablespoons vodka (optional)

1 tablespoon vanilla extract

Stevia to equal 4 teaspoons sugar (optional)

1 Combine all the ingredients in a blender, and blend until smooth. Refrigerate until cold.

2 Pour the chilled mixture into your ice cream maker and churn until thick.

COOK'S NOTE: *Clear spirits like vodka and white wine are the only two alcoholic beverages recommended on the strict version of the Plan. Adding vodka to sorbet improves its texture. Use very ripe organic strawberries for this; conventional berries hold onto pesticides. Only add the stevia if your strawberries are not super sweet.*

"One of the first things I teach in therapy to all of my clients is orienting, connecting to the environment through the senses. We get most of our information through our eyes. So typically my first invitation is let your eyes go where they want to go. What do you notice around you? Imagine if you weren't in the driver's seat and your eyes could just roam around, what would they be attracted to? Where would they get stuck? What are they curious about? This moves our attention from an internal experience to an external experience. And the more we do that, the more our nervous system settles down."

MAHSHID FASHANDI HAGER, LMFT, SEP

PER SERVING: 1g protein, 6g carbohydrates, 6g fat, 5g saturated fat, 8mg sodium, 113mg potassium, 1g fiber

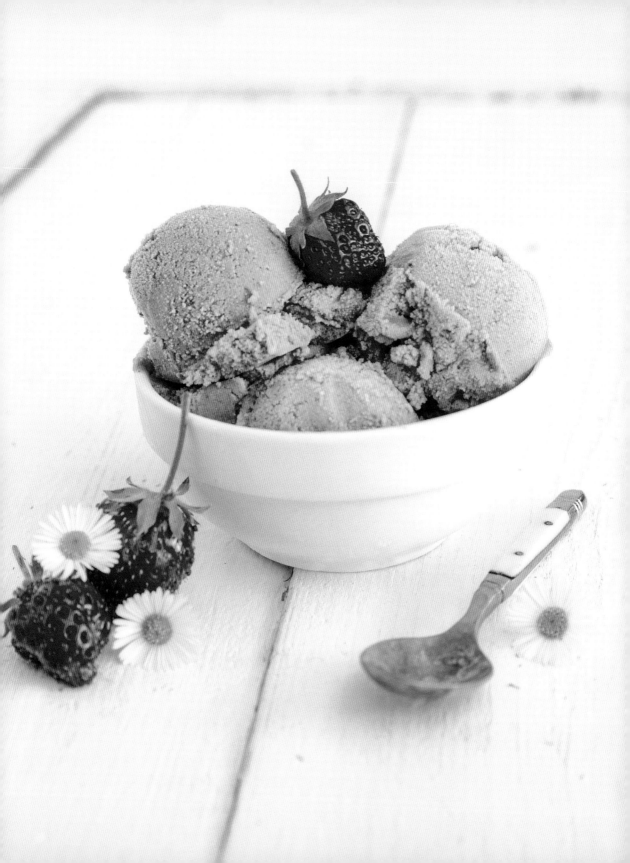

Choco-Berry Sorbet

I developed this dessert out of desperation for ice cream. You won't believe anything so rich and tasty is dairy- and sugar-free! Impress last-minute dinner guests by creating this in less than 5 minutes. People won't believe there's no chocolate in it.

Makes 4 servings

Prep time: N/A
Cooking time: 5 minutes
Passive time: N/A

Budget friendly: Very

2 cups (275g) frozen strawberries, blueberries, or blackberries

½ cup room-temperature Creamy Not-ella Butter (p. 28)

1 Place the fruit in a food processor fitted with the S-blade and process just until the sound gets quieter and pieces are uniformly small.

2 Add the Creamy Not-ella Butter and process just until smooth.

3 Scoop and serve right away. This does not freeze well. Leftover sorbet can be refrigerated and used the next day as the base for a smoothie.

PER ⅓-CUP SERVING (with frozen strawberries):
6g protein, 15g carbohydrates, 8g fat, 3g saturated fat, 51mg sodium, 222mg potassium, 5g fiber

Sunbutter Freezer Fudge

Where do I get my recipe ideas? I taste something somewhere, I see a recipe online, and sometimes it's from a request. When a reader requested a fudge-like treat, I adapted a recipe I'd received from a functional-medicine nutritionist. This tastes like a cross between fudge and a peanut butter cup.

Makes 16 squares

Prep time: 5 minutes
Cooking time: 2 minutes
Passive time: 60 minutes

Budget friendly: Very

⅔ cup (170g) no-salt-added sunflower seed butter

½ cup (125mL) extra-virgin coconut oil

2 tablespoons unsweetened carob powder

2 teaspoons vanilla extract

Stevia to equal 8 teaspoons sugar

1 Heat all the ingredients in a saucepan over low heat, stirring until smooth, or microwave on 50% power for 60 to 90 seconds, stirring once.

2 Spoon into silicone molds, ice cube trays, or an 8 × 8-inch baking dish lined with parchment paper.

3 Freeze until firm, at least 60 minutes.

4 Pop out of the molds or ice cube trays or remove from dish and cut into 16 squares. Store in the freezer in a freezer-safe zip-top bag or glass container.

COOK'S NOTE: *Best made in silicone candy molds or ice cube trays, so you can pop the pieces out easily. These get very soft at room temperature, so don't take them far from the freezer.*

PER 1½-INCH × 1½-INCH SQUARE (with salted sunbutter):
2g protein, 3g carbohydrates, 11g fat, 1g saturated fat, 40mg sodium, 6mg potassium, 2g fiber

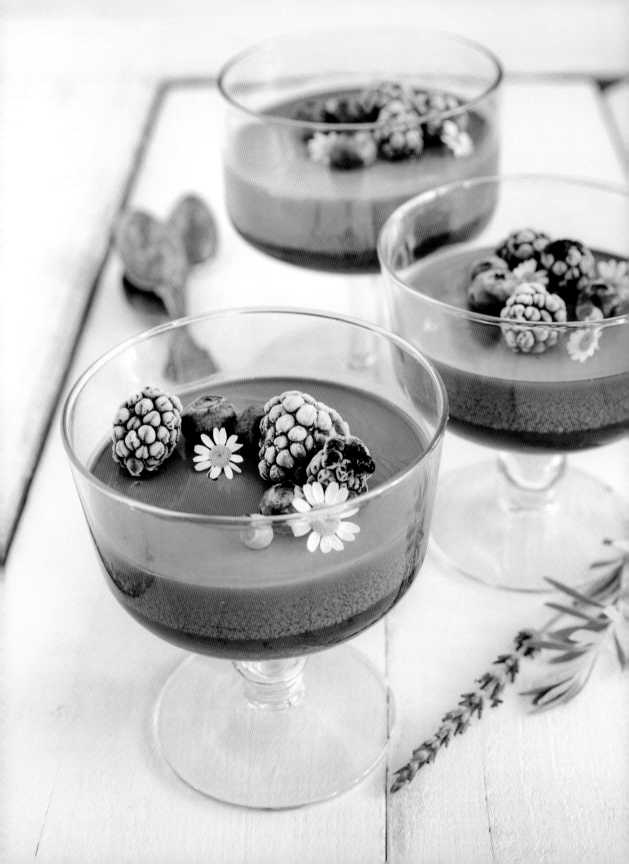

Fruit Juice Gelatin

One tester reported coming home and finding her husband standing in front of the fridge eating this delicious low-carb dessert right out of the trays.

Makes 8 servings

Prep time: N/A
Cooking time: 5 minutes
Passive time: 1½ hours

Budget friendly: Very

2 cups (500mL) blackberry juice or any Plan-friendly juice blend (see Cook's Note)

1 tablespoon grass-fed gelatin

1 cup (250mL) canned light or regular coconut milk

Stevia to equal 4 teaspoons sugar

1 Stir the gelatin into the juice a little at a time in a medium saucepan.

2 Heat over medium heat for five minutes, stirring frequently, until the gelatin completely dissolves.

3 Remove from the heat and stir in the coconut milk and stevia.

4 Pour into a square glass baking dish, individual dessert cups, oiled ice cube trays, or silicone candy or baking molds.

5 Chill until firm, about 1½ hours. Store in the refrigerator covered in plastic wrap.

COOK'S NOTE: *Gelatin provides many health benefits and may be especially helpful for migraine brains. It's important to order grass-fed gelatin from healthy, properly raised animals. Choose 100% fruit juice that contains no added sugars or triggers (pretty much all are made from concentrate). If you have a juicer, create your own juice from your favorite Plan-friendly fruits and sweeter vegetables.*

PER SERVING: 2g protein, 5g carbohydrates, 2g fat, 1g saturated fat, 9mg sodium, 84mg potassium, 0g fiber

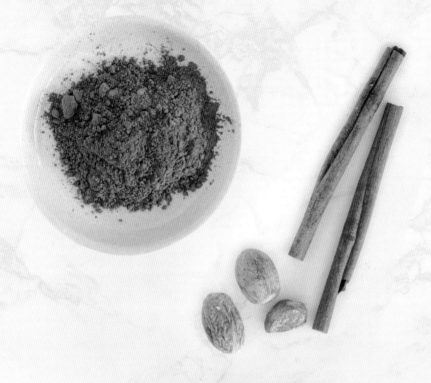

"A big part of the resilience journey for me is humility. As resilient as I am and as tough as I am, my ego loves to tell me I can handle everything and anything and that I should pick up more. I've told myself this story about how I was born for all this challenge. That is not helpful. The world doesn't need me to be a martyr and the world doesn't need me to break myself at the expense of whatever this is."

ABBY MASLIN, AUTHOR OF *LOVE YOU HARD: A MEMOIR OF MARRIAGE, BRAIN INJURY, AND REINVENTING LOVE*

"Resilience is the ability to move forward. In the grief space, we never 'move on,' we move forward. I'm not 'over' my husband or our marriage or the life we had. I still feel that he's with me and still very much a part of our lives. That is resilience and it's something I'm so grateful for."

MELISSA GOULD, AUTHOR OF *WIDOWISH*

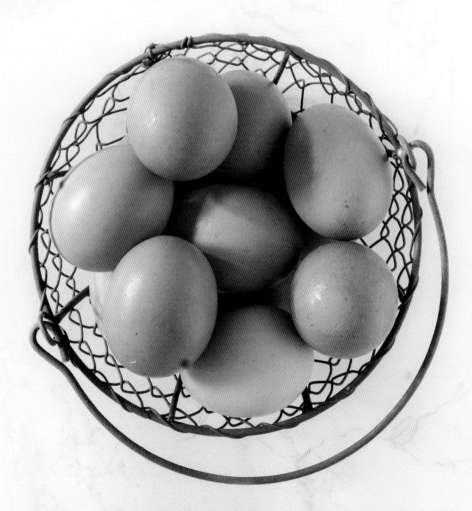

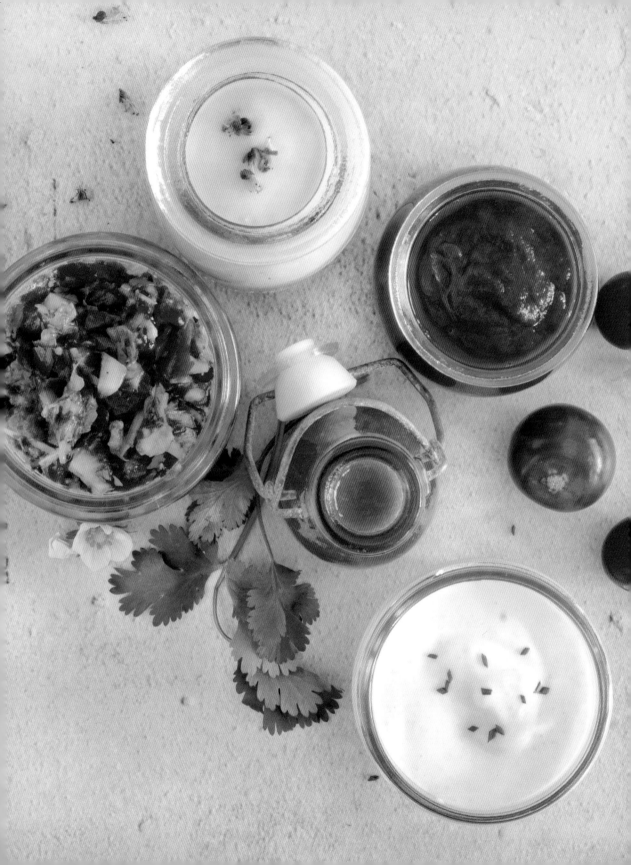

Sauces, Condiments, and Basics

Most store-bought dressings and condiments include trigger ingredients or are too high in sugar or sodium. It's important to have dressings, sauces, and condiments on hand for flavor and enjoyment. Many of the recipes that follow are called for in other recipes throughout the book. I love having freshly made salad dressing ready to go, a variety of salsas to enjoy with chips, and condiments for burgers. Don't miss the recipes for vegetable broth, a quick pizza crust, and gravy near the end!

Cherry-Sesame Dressing

....

Makes ½ cup

Prep time:	5 minutes
Cooking time:	N/A
Passive time:	N/A

....

Budget friendly: Very

¼ cup (60mL) unsweetened cherry juice

2 tablespoons tahini

1 tablespoon honey

1 tablespoon minced fresh ginger

1 teaspoon white vinegar

1 teaspoon dark toasted sesame oil

⅛ teaspoon white pepper

1 Place all the ingredients in a blender and blend until very smooth, stopping to scrape down the sides as needed.

COOK'S NOTE: *Find tahini (finely ground sesame paste) in most larger grocery stores, natural foods markets, or online.*

 If rice wine vinegar is not a trigger for you, use it in place of the white vinegar. If coconut aminos are not a trigger for you, add a splash to make the dressing less sweet.

PER 1-TABLESPOON SERVING:
1g protein, 6g carbohydrates, 3g fat, 1g saturated fat, 0mg sodium, 62mg potassium, 0g fiber

Mango-Jalapeño Dressing

....

Makes ½ cup

Prep time:	5 minutes
Cooking time:	N/A
Passive time:	30 minutes

....

Budget friendly: Very

¼–1 jalapeño pepper, stemmed and seeded

1 small or ½ large ripe mango, peeled and seeded

1 tablespoon mayonnaise

½ teaspoon white vinegar

2 tablespoons extra-virgin olive oil

6 tablespoons (90mL) filtered water

1 Place all the ingredients, starting with one quarter of the jalapeño, in a blender and blend until very smooth, stopping to scrape down the sides as needed.

2 Let sit for at least 30 minutes, then taste. If desired, add more jalapeño. Keep refrigerated and use within 5 days.

COOK'S NOTE: *The mangoes provide the acidity needed for a salad dressing, as vinegar is limited on the Plan until you have tested it.*

PER 1-TABLESPOON SERVING:
0g protein, 5g carbohydrates, 5g fat, 1g saturated fat, 11mg sodium, 4mg potassium, 1g fiber

Shallot-Mustard Vinaigrette ⊘ ⊘ ⊘ ⊘

Makes about ½ cup

Prep time: 5 minutes
Cooking time: N/A
Passive time: N/A

Budget friendly: Very

1 teaspoon minced shallot, soaked in ice water for 10 minutes and drained

5 cherry tomatoes

¼ cup (60mL) extra-virgin olive oil

1 tablespoon filtered water

1 teaspoon white vinegar

1 teaspoon dry mustard

½ teaspoon dried thyme

1 Blend all the ingredients until very smooth, stopping to scrape down the sides as needed.

2 Store in a clean glass jar in the refrigerator.

COOK'S NOTE: *This makes an excellent marinade for grilled vegetables or meat. A small blender like a Nutribullet works well for this recipe.*

PER 1-TABLESPOON SERVING:
1g protein, 2g carbohydrates, 6g fat, 1g saturated fat, 3mg sodium, 137mg potassium, 0g fiber

"When I was in fix-it mode, underneath that was a feeling that I was broken in some way. As if there was something wrong with me because I had an illness that needed to be 'fixed.' What I started to realize was, 'Oh, I'm trying to *go back to normal*, because I think if I'm healthy, then I won't be broken.' I realized that I needed to focus on optimal health. How do I find my optimal health with my particular physiology, my limitations, and what my body needs? That opened up this whole world. And the sense of relief started, like setting down rocks off my shoulders. I'm not broken. I just have to live my life differently."

**KIMBERLY JOY,
WRITER AND LUPUS PATIENT**

Chunky Tomato Sauce

Makes 4 cups

Prep time: 5 minutes
Cooking time: 15 minutes
Passive time: N/A

Budget friendly: Very

1 tablespoon extra-virgin olive oil

2 shallots, minced

2 cloves garlic, minced

1 (28-ounce [800g]) can no-salt-added diced tomatoes

1 teaspoon dried oregano

½ teaspoon freshly ground black pepper

¼ cup (5g) chopped fresh basil

1 Heat the oil over medium heat in a medium-size nonstick or cast-iron pan until shimmering.

2 Sauté the shallots and garlic for 2 minutes.

3 Add the tomatoes, oregano, and pepper and bring just to a boil.

4 Reduce heat and simmer uncovered for 10 minutes.

5 Remove from the heat and stir in the basil.

PER ¼-CUP SERVING:
2g protein, 11g carbohydrates, 4g fat, 1g saturated fat, 28mg sodium, 48mg potassium, 2g fiber

Cranberry-Pear Sauce

Makes 2 cups

Prep time: 5 minutes
Cooking time: 20 minutes
Passive time: N/A

Budget friendly: Very

2 pears, peeled, cored, cut into chunks

10 ounces (285g) fresh or frozen and thawed cranberries

Stevia to equal 6 teaspoons sugar

1 Place all the ingredients in a food processor and pulse until chunky and the cranberries are broken up.

2 Pour into a saucepan. Heat until just boiling, then reduce heat and simmer, partially covered, for 15 minutes.

3 Let cool, then taste and add more stevia if needed.

COOK'S NOTE: *Sweeter pears will require less stevia. This can be made 2 days ahead of a holiday. It freezes beautifully.*

PER 2-TABLESPOON SERVING:
0g protein, 7g carbohydrates, 0g fat, 0g saturated fat, 1mg sodium, 48mg potassium, 2g fiber

Taqueria-Style Faux Guacamole

Makes 1½ cups

Prep time:	5 minutes
Cooking time:	N/A
Passive time:	N/A

Budget friendly: Very

2 Mexican squash (200–220g), ends trimmed, quartered (see Cook's Note)

1 jalapeño pepper, stemmed, roughly chopped

2 cloves garlic

¼ cup (12–15g) cilantro, roughly chopped

⅛ teaspoon salt

2 tablespoons extra-virgin olive or filtered extra-virgin coconut oil, melted

1 Begin with all the ingredients at room temperature. Add the squash, jalapeño, garlic, cilantro, and salt to a food processor. Pulse until it reaches a creamy and smooth consistency.

2 Turn on food processor and add the oil in a slow stream.

COOK'S NOTE: *Since avocados are not on the Plan until you've tested them, this sauce might fill that need. Frequently served in taco shops in place of guacamole, it's great with tortilla chips, spread on burgers, or as the base for a chimichurri-style sauce for meat or fish—just add parsley. It could also be a flavor-enhancer for leftovers. Mix it into a pan with cooked rice, diced chicken, and a splash of water. Mexican squash, also called gray squash, looks like speckled, pale green zucchini. Denser and more bulbous, it's required for this recipe. Find it at Latin markets. If you can tolerate more salt, use ¼ teaspoon for this recipe.*

"If you can have an optimistic perspective, studies show that that makes a huge difference in developing your own resilience. I think that there's a spiritual element to it, whatever you believe in. Maybe it's just practicing gratitude, maybe it's meditation."

MADDY DYCHTWALD, CO-FOUNDER, AGE WAVE

 If limes are not a trigger for you, add a squeeze.

PER 2-TABLESPOON SERVING:
0g protein, 1g carbohydrates, 2g fat, 0g saturated fat, 26mg sodium, 44mg potassium, 0g fiber

Mango Salsa

Makes 2 cups

Prep time: 10 minutes
Cooking time: N/A
Passive time: 30 minutes

Budget friendly: Very

1 ripe mango, diced medium

1 pint (285g) cherry tomatoes, diced medium

1 small carrot, diced medium

1 red bell pepper, diced medium

1 jalapeño pepper, stemmed, seeded, and minced (or to taste)

1 tablespoon Hot Sauce (p. 196)

½ teaspoon white vinegar

¼ teaspoon white pepper

2 cups (100g) minced cilantro (optional)

1 Mix all the ingredients in a bowl.

2 Let sit at least 30 minutes before serving.

COOK'S NOTE: *If you do not like raw carrots in salsa, substitute another mango or a ripe peach or nectarine. Substitute Chile Pepper Sauce (p. 267, The Migraine Relief Plan) for the Hot Sauce.*

 If you have tested them, one diced avocado and the juice of one lime are excellent additions.

PER 2-TABLESPOON SERVING:
1g protein, 4g carbohydrates, 0g fat, 0g saturated fat, 33mg sodium, 196mg potassium, 1g fiber

Salsa Fresca

Makes 2 cups

Prep time: 10 minutes
Cooking time: N/A
Passive time: N/A

Budget friendly: Very

1.25 pounds (575g) cherry tomatoes

2 hot red peppers, seeded

2 green onions, snipped into pieces

2 cloves garlic

2 cups packed (100g) cilantro

1 teaspoon cumin (optional)

1 Put all the ingredients in a food processor and pulse 15 times, scraping down the sides after every 5 pulses.

2 Store in a clean glass container up to 5 days.

COOK'S NOTE: *You can use any variety of hot pepper; ask at the store about heat levels. Store-bought cherry tomatoes are the most reliably flavorful tomatoes you can buy at the grocery. Use home-grown or farmers' market tomatoes when available.*

PER 2-TABLESPOON SERVING:
1g protein, 2g carbohydrates, 0g fat, 0g saturated fat, 4mg sodium, 120mg potassium, 0g fiber

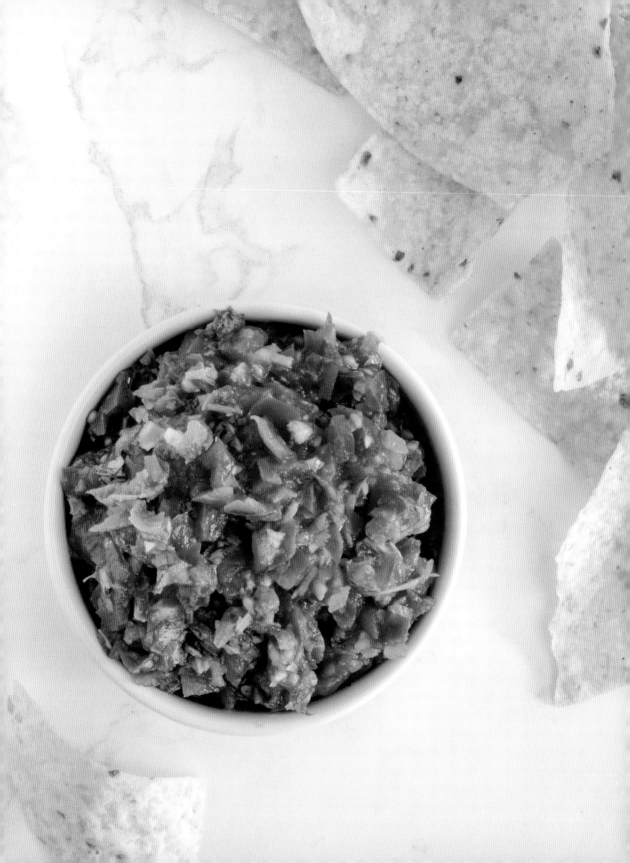

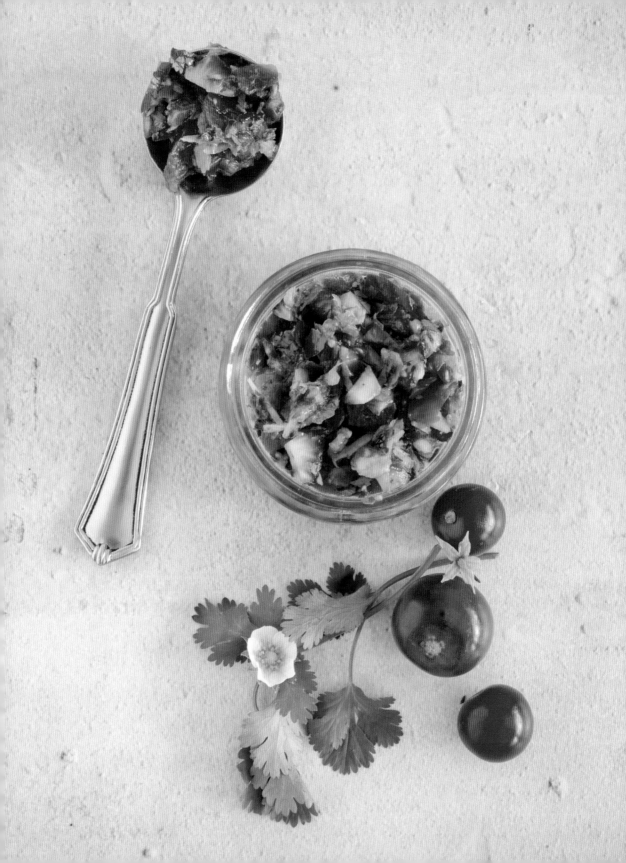

Strawberry Salsa

Makes about 2 cups

Prep time: 10 minutes
Cooking time: N/A
Passive time: N/A

Budget friendly: Very

1 cup (145g) strawberries, hulled

1 pint (285g) cherry tomatoes

1–2 jalapeño peppers (or to taste), seeded

1 green onion, roughly chopped

1 handful cilantro (optional)

1 teaspoon white vinegar

⅛ teaspoon white pepper

1 Put all the ingredients in a food processor and pulse 15 times, scraping down the sides after every 5 pulses.

2 Let salsa sit at least 30 minutes before serving.

COOK'S NOTE: *Serve with chips or place atop grilled fish, chicken, or pork. Buy the ripest tomatoes available. Omit the cilantro if you hate it. Use red jalapeño peppers when in season.*

 If white balsamic vinegar is not a trigger for you, substitute that for the white vinegar.

"Resilience is about being able to construct a new meaning for yourself in the face of all of that loss. To be able to say, 'Okay, I thought my satisfaction in life was going to come from taking hikes and being the capable, active person who could get anything done. So how do I construct a sense of myself and a sense of my life where I can still feel like I'm contributing? Where can I still feel like there's meaning and value?'"

JULIE REHMEYER, AUTHOR OF *THROUGH THE SHADOWLANDS: A SCIENCE WRITER'S JOURNEY INTO AN ILLNESS SCIENCE DOESN'T UNDERSTAND*

PER 2-TABLESPOON SERVING: 0g protein, 2g carbohydrates, 0g fat, 0g saturated fat, 1mg sodium, 66mg potassium, 1g fiber

Egg-Free Mayonnaise

Makes about 1 cup

Prep time: 5 minutes
Cooking time: N/A
Passive time: N/A

Budget friendly: Very

1 (15.5-ounce [450g]) can no-salt-added chickpeas (not drained, see Cook's Note)

1½ teaspoons white vinegar

1½ teaspoons dry mustard

¼ teaspoon fine sea salt

Stevia to equal 1 teaspoon sugar

⅛ teaspoon cream of tartar (optional)

¾ cup (175mL) light olive oil

1 Pour most of the chickpea liquid into a container. Then pour ¼ cup of the thickest liquid from the bottom of the can into a large glass measuring cup or jar that your immersion blender fits into. Reserve chickpeas and remaining liquid for another use.

2 Add the vinegar, mustard, salt, stevia, and cream of tartar (if using).

3 Using an immersion blender, blend until white and fluffy, about 1 minute.

4 With the blender running, drizzle in the oil in a slow, thin stream, over 4 to 5 minutes.

5 Refrigerate and use within a week. The mixture will emulsify and thicken as it chills.

COOK'S NOTE: *Chickpea liquid is the only bean liquid that will work in this recipe. You must use an immersion blender for this recipe, and light olive oil (not the good stuff). Some testers decreased the amount of mustard to reduce the spiciness.*

"Getting sick with vestibular migraine, I was able to take a step back, realize what's important and reflect on what my new road and journey was going to be like. And honestly, that came through getting a counselor. I sought help because I knew I wasn't able to do this alone. And I knew that I needed someone to help me shift my mindset. I ended up quitting my job to work from home, to find conditions that worked for me."

KAYLA MCCAIN, VEDA PATIENT ADVOCATE AND VESTIBULAR MIGRAINE BLOGGER, *TRUE KAYLAISMS*

PER 1-TABLESPOON SERVING: 0g protein, 0g carbohydrates, 11g fat, 2g saturated fat, 33mg sodium, 0mg potassium, 0g fiber

Olive Oil Mayonnaise

Makes 2 cups

Prep time: 5–9 minutes
Cooking time: N/A
Passive time: 2 hours

Budget friendly: Very

Allow all ingredients to come to room temperature, about two hours, before beginning this recipe.

1 egg

1 egg yolk

1 tablespoon distilled white vinegar

1 tablespoon filtered water

1 cup (250mL) light olive oil, divided

½ teaspoon dry mustard

¼ teaspoon sea salt, pulverized

¼ teaspoon cream of tartar (optional)

1 slice cucumber, peeled and chopped (optional)

> If pickles and apple cider vinegar are not triggers for you, use 1 pickle and apple cider vinegar in place of the cucumber and distilled white vinegar.

Hand/immersion blender instructions:

1 Place the egg, yolk, vinegar, water, ¼ cup of the olive oil, mustard, sea salt, cream of tartar (if using), and cucumber (if using) in a large glass measuring cup or jar that your immersion blender fits into.

2 Blend with an immersion blender for about 1 minute.

3 With the blender running, drizzle in the remaining oil in a slow, thin stream, stopping when the mixture is the consistency of store-bought mayonnaise.

4 Refrigerate and eat within a week.

Blender instructions:

1 Place the egg, yolk, vinegar, water, ¼ cup of the olive oil, mustard, sea salt, cream of tartar (if using), and cucumber (if using) in the blender.

2 Blend for 1 minute on high.

3 With the blender running on high, drizzle in the remaining oil in a slow, thin stream. This may take up to 2 to 3 minutes; pay attention to the sound the blender is making and the look of the mayo. Stop once it is thick and creamy.

4 Transfer to a clean glass jar. Refrigerate and eat within a week.

COOK'S NOTE: *Use pasteurized eggs for the safest mayonnaise. Use less-expensive and milder tasting light olive oil for this recipe. Do not use dark extra-virgin. The cream of tartar helps maintain the emulsion, but omit it if you are sensitive to it. Do not attempt mayonnaise when a thunderstorm threatens or is in progress as it won't bind. You don't need to add all of the oil; stop once the mayonnaise is nice and thick. If you break the mayonnaise emulsion, The Joy of Cooking suggests these two fixes: 1) Blend in 1 teaspoon of warm water. 2) Put another egg yolk in a clean bowl and very, very slowly beat the broken emulsion into the yolk.*

PER 1-TABLESPOON SERVING: 0g protein, 0g carbohydrates, 7g fat, 1g saturated fat, 21mg sodium, 8mg potassium, 0g fiber

Hot Sauce

Makes 1 cup

Prep time: 10 minutes
Cooking time: 25 minutes
Passive time: N/A

Budget friendly: Very

¾ cup (180mL) filtered water

1 medium red bell pepper, stemmed, seeded, cut into chunks

1 habanero pepper or 2 red jalapeños, seeded

1 teaspoon white distilled vinegar

Stevia to equal up to 4 teaspoons sugar (optional)

1 Place the water, peppers, and vinegar in a small saucepan and bring to a boil.

2 Reduce heat and simmer for 20 minutes. Let cool.

3 Process in a blender until very smooth, adding stevia to your taste if desired. Transfer to clean glass jars and store in the refrigerator.

COOK'S NOTE: *Green jalapeños will taste fine, but they will muddy the color of the sauce. Red jalapeños may only be available in the summer months. Substitute 4 teaspoons coconut sugar for the stevia if you wish.*

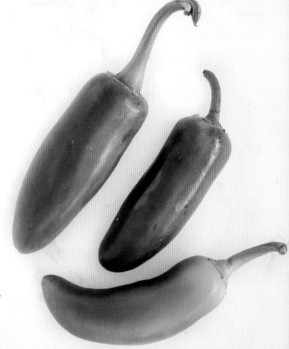

PER 1-TEASPOON SERVING: 0g protein, 0g carbohydrates, 0g fat, 0g saturated fat, 0mg sodium, 4mg potassium, 0g fiber

Ketchup

Makes 1½ cups

Prep time: 10 minutes
Cooking time: 1¼–1½ hours
Passive time: N/A

Budget friendly: Very

1 tablespoon extra-virgin olive oil

6 green onions, white parts only, roughly chopped

1 clove garlic, minced

1 (14.5-ounce [450g]) can no-salt-added tomato puree or tomato pieces

¼ cup (40g) coconut sugar

2 tablespoons distilled white vinegar

¼ teaspoon ground mustard

Pinch ground cloves

 If apple cider, balsamic, or white balsamic vinegars are not a trigger for you, substitute one of them for the white vinegar.

1 Heat the olive oil over medium heat in a deep, heavy-bottomed saucepan or pot, then add the onions. Cook about 9 minutes until onions are translucent and starting to caramelize, stirring occasionally. Add the garlic and cook 1 minute.

2 Add the remaining ingredients and bring to a bubble, stirring. Reduce the heat until just barely simmering. Cook for 60 minutes, partially covered, stirring every 15 minutes. When uncovering the pot to stir, blot condensation from inside the lid with a kitchen towel.

3 Place mixture in a blender and blend until completely smooth. If ketchup is not thick enough, put it back into the pot and continue to cook on low for another 15 to 30 minutes, until it reaches the desired consistency. Use a funnel to pour into clean glass bottles.

4 Refrigerate and use within a month. The flavor develops as it chills.

COOK'S NOTE: *Reserve the green parts of the onions for making Low-Sodium Chicken Broth (p. 136) or Beany-Brothy Deliciousness (p. 142). A regular blender will produce a smoother consistency, but an immersion blender works fine.*

PER 1-TABLESPOON SERVING: 0g protein, 3g carbohydrates, 0g fat, 0g saturated fat, 34mg sodium, 75mg potassium, 0g fiber

Thai Curry Paste (Green and Red)

Makes 1 cup

Prep time:	15 minutes
Cooking time:	N/A
Passive time:	N/A

Budget friendly: Moderate

1 cup (55g) chopped cilantro stems, from 1 bunch

6 cloves garlic, roughly chopped

1 (2-inch) piece (60g) fresh ginger root, peeled and roughly chopped

2 large or 4 small shallots, roughly chopped

3 stems fresh lemongrass (see Cook's Note)

4 large hot chile peppers (green or red), seeded and roughly chopped

1 tablespoon turmeric (only if making red curry paste)

1–3 tablespoons filtered water

1 Place all the ingredients in a food processor or blender. Add just enough filtered water to blend into a fine paste.

2 Freeze the unused portion in small containers for later. Ice cube trays work great for this, so you can thaw only the amount you need.

COOK'S NOTE: *Reserve cilantro tops for another recipe, like Carrot-Ginger Soup (p. 74). To prepare lemongrass, peel off the outer hard leaves, then finely slice just the soft end near the bulb and discard the rest. If you cannot find fresh lemongrass, substitute 1 tablespoon dried lemongrass soaked in 2 tablespoons hot filtered water for at least 30 minutes. Add the lemongrass water to the recipe in place of the filtered water. Include the ribs and seeds from the chiles for a hotter chile paste. Chile fumes can be strong while blending.*

ADD TO: *Quick and Easy Ramen (p. 69), Twice-Baked Thai-Spiced Potatoes (p. 84), Coconut-Curried Greens (p. 110), Thai-Style Chicken Soup (p. 138), and Thai-Style Shrimp Curry (p. 153).*

PER 1-TABLESPOON SERVING: 0g protein, 3g carbohydrates, 1g fat, 0g saturated fat, 2mg sodium, 1mg potassium, 0g fiber

Garam Masala

Makes a little more than ¼ cup

Prep time: 5 minutes
Cooking time: N/A
Passive time: N/A

Budget friendly: Moderate
(if you have to buy the spices)

2 teaspoons cumin seeds

2 teaspoons fenugreek seeds

2 teaspoons mustard seeds

2 teaspoons cardamom
seed pods

2 teaspoons fennel seeds

1 Toast all the ingredients in a dry pan over medium-low heat for 3 to 5 minutes to bring out the flavor. Allow to cool.

2 Transfer the spice mixture to an electric spice grinder. Blend into a powder. Store in a clean glass jar.

ADD TO: *Carrot-Ginger Soup (p. 74), South Asian-Inspired Chickpea Masala (p. 86), Coconut-Curried Greens (p. 110), Curried Roast Cauliflower (p. 115), or Cauliflower-Chickpea Curry (p. 150).*

"Advocacy gave me back the power that chronic migraine stole from me. It changed me and I'm grateful. Advocacy can take many forms. You can talk to your senators during Headache on the Hill or run a 5k with Miles for Migraine. You can advocate for yourself by educating yourself. You can advocate by sharing something on social media and making your family and friends aware."

KATIE GOLDEN, *GOLDEN GRAINE*

Greek Spice Blend

Makes about 2 tablespoons

Prep time: 5 minutes
Cooking time: N/A
Passive time: N/A

Budget friendly: Moderate

1 tablespoon toasted sesame seeds, cooled

1 teaspoon dried spearmint

1 teaspoon dried oregano

1 teaspoon dried thyme

½ teaspoon sea salt (optional)

1 Place all the ingredients in an electric spice grinder. Blend into a powder. Store in a clean glass jar.

COOK'S NOTE: *To toast sesame seeds, place in a dry skillet over medium heat and cook, shaking the pan frequently, until medium brown.*

ADD TO: *Herbed Olive Oil Crackers (p. 31), Quickie Microwave Egg Scramble (p. 39), Mediterranean Tuna Burgers (p. 70), Lazy Chicken (p. 90), Sheet Pan Chicken Thighs (p. 89), Easy Roasted Potatoes (p. 148), Sweet Potato Oven Fries (p. 113), or Curried Roast Cauliflower (p. 115).*

Pumpkin Pie Spice

Makes slightly more than ⅓ cup

Prep time: 5 minutes
Cooking time: N/A
Passive time: N/A

Budget friendly: Moderate

2 teaspoons ground cinnamon

2 teaspoons ground ginger

1 teaspoon ground nutmeg

½ teaspoon ground cloves

½ teaspoon ground cardamom

1 Mix all the ingredients thoroughly and store in a clean glass jar.

ADD TO: *Trail Mix (p. 22), Pumpkin-Spice Waffles (p. 46), Carrot-Ginger Soup (p. 74), Sweet Potato Oven Fries (p. 113), Pumpkin Risotto (p. 121), Pumpkin Pie (p. 166), or Apple-Spice Mug Cake (p. 167).*

"Beauty hunting is a spiritual practice and a way of being in the world. Some people walk around and look for things to be irritated, annoyed, and frustrated by. I don't want to live like that. That's not to say I don't get irritated, annoyed, and frustrated. I'm human, but I'd rather orient myself to the beauty. Sometimes you have to look harder and reevaluate, redefine, and completely change what you thought beauty is and was and does. For me, it's a way of being present. It anchors me to being here. To stopping. What are five beautiful things, right here, right now?"

JENNIFER PASTILOFF, AUTHOR OF
ON BEING HUMAN

Seafood Seasoning

Makes about ½ cup

Prep time:	5 minutes
Cooking time:	N/A
Passive time:	N/A

Budget friendly: Moderate

5 bay leaves, crunched
5 green cardamom pods
½ teaspoon celery seed
½ teaspoon black peppercorns
½ teaspoon red pepper flakes
1 teaspoon garlic powder
1 teaspoon dry mustard
½ teaspoon ground nutmeg
½ teaspoon cayenne
½ teaspoon ground allspice
½ teaspoon mace (optional)

1 Place the bay leaves, green cardamom pods, celery seed, black peppercorns, and red pepper flakes in an electric spice grinder. Blend into a powder, stopping every minute or so to check on your progress. The cardamom pods may not completely pulverize.

2 Add the remaining spices and blend until one color.

3 Sift through a fine mesh strainer before storing in a clean glass jar.

ADD TO: *Honey-Mustard Salmon Salad (p. 63), Grilled Salmon (p. 65), or Tuna-Rice Salad (p. 62).*

COOK'S NOTE: *Mace is the outer, lacy covering of nutmeg seeds. Include if you want to achieve a flavor similar to the store-bought seasoning from Maryland.*

Spice Rub for Red Meat

Makes about ⅔ cup

Prep time: 5 minutes
Cooking time: N/A
Passive time: N/A

Budget friendly: Moderate (to buy the spices)

2 teaspoons ground cumin

2 teaspoons smoked paprika

2 teaspoons freshly cracked black pepper

2 teaspoons garlic powder

2 teaspoons dried tomato powder (optional)

½ teaspoon chipotle powder

1 Mix all the ingredients together until one color. Store in a clean glass jar.

ADD TO: *Beef Barbacoa (p. 102) in place of the dry-rub mixture in that recipe.*

COOK'S NOTE: *Makes enough for 6 pork chops or 2 to 4 steaks, depending on their size. Dried tomato powder is worth ordering from an online marketplace, as it caramelizes the spice rub onto the meat.*

Taco Seasoning

Makes just about ½ cup

Prep time: 5 minutes
Cooking time: N/A
Passive time: N/A

Budget friendly: Moderate

1 tablespoon mild chili powder

1½ teaspoons ground cumin

1 teaspoon freshly ground black pepper

½ teaspoon garlic powder

½ teaspoon smoked paprika

¼ teaspoon dried oregano

¼ teaspoon cayenne pepper (optional)

1 Mix all the ingredients thoroughly and store in a clean glass jar.

ADD TO: *Tex-Mex Migas (p. 50), Quinrizo Taco Salad (p. 66), Quick Turkey Tacos (p. 98), Sweet Potato Oven Fries (p. 113), Quick Bean Tacos (p. 146), or Tex-Mex Skillet Dinner (p. 156).*

Gluten-Free Flour Blend

Makes 4 cups

Prep time: 5 minutes
Cooking time: N/A
Passive time: N/A

Budget friendly: Moderate

1 cup (120g) gluten-free oat flour

1 cup (135g) sweet sorghum flour

1 cup (160g) brown rice flour

1 cup (120g) tapioca flour

4 teaspoons psyllium husk fiber

1 Whisk together the ingredients. Store in an airtight container.

COOK'S NOTE: *Tapioca flour is also called tapioca starch. You can substitute millet flour for sorghum flour in this blend. If you have a high-speed blender, make your own oat flour from gluten-free rolled oats, grinding as finely as possible. Substitute this cup for cup for wheat flour when converting any baking recipe, but note that if the batter or dough seems too dry, you'll need to add more liquid than called for in the original recipe to match the texture of the batter or dough. Gluten-free flour absorbs much more moisture than wheat flour.*

"The biggest mistake I made for so long was trying to recapture the life that I had lost. Nothing else was acceptable to me. And with a lot of time, I started moving toward acceptance: It is what it is. I could see that if I was looking for that other life, I would probably be 85 and still looking."

CYNTHIA TOUSSAINT, AUTHOR OF *BATTLE FOR GRACE: A MEMOIR OF PAIN, REDEMPTION, AND IMPOSSIBLE LOVE*

Low-Sodium Vegetable Broth

Makes 12 cups

Prep time: 15 minutes
Cooking time: 2½ hours
Passive time: N/A

Budget friendly: Very

2 tablespoons extra-virgin olive oil

2 large leeks, cleaned and roughly chopped

6 cloves garlic, smashed

3 carrots, roughly chopped

3 celery stalks, roughly chopped

8 ounces (225g) shiitake mushrooms, cleaned and roughly chopped

½ teaspoon sea salt (optional)

½ cup (125mL) white wine (optional)

3 bay leaves

12 cups (3L) filtered water

1 Heat the oil in a large stockpot or Dutch oven over medium heat.

2 Sauté all the vegetables until golden brown. Sprinkle with the salt, if using.

3 Pour the white wine (or ½ cup of filtered water if not using wine) into the pan. Use a wooden spoon to deglaze the pan by scraping up any brown bits. Cook until most of the liquid is gone.

4 Add the bay leaves to the pot along with the filtered water.

5 Bring just to a boil, then reduce the heat, cover, and simmer for 2 hours.

6 Let cool for 15 minutes, then put in the refrigerator to cool overnight to deepen the flavor.

7 Strain the vegetables and store the broth in clean jars. Dispose of or compost the vegetables. Refrigerate the broth and use within 5 days, or freeze in freezer-safe jars or zip-top gallon freezer bags for up to six months.

COOK'S NOTE: *If you have frozen leek tops from another dish, toss in whatever you have. If using frozen or pre-cleaned leeks, you'll need 2 cups sliced (200g). You can omit the salt for the lowest-sodium version. If you can't find shiitake mushrooms, use creminis.*

PER 1-CUP SERVING (with ½ teaspoon sea salt):
1g protein, 6g carbohydrates, 2g fat, 0g saturated fat, 135mg sodium (36mg without added salt), 213mg potassium, 2g fiber

Quick Pizza Crust

Makes 1 crust (6 servings)

Prep time: 5 minutes
Cooking time: 13 minutes
Passive time: 30 minutes

Budget friendly: Very

1 cup (250mL) filtered water

1 cup (130g) chickpea flour

2 tablespoons extra-virgin olive oil, divided

2 tablespoons no-salt-added Italian seasoning

1 teaspoon garlic powder

1 Preheat the oven to 450°F (230°C), setting one rack in the center and one under the broiler. Place a 12-inch cast-iron pan in the oven to heat.

2 Blend the water, flour, 1 tablespoon of the olive oil, and the spices in a blender until smooth. Let stand 30 minutes.

3 When the oven reaches temperature, remove the pan carefully with hot pads. Add the remaining oil, swirling the pan to coat evenly up the sides.

4 Pour the batter into the pan.

5 Bake for 8 minutes on the center rack, until edges are crispy and center is set.

COOK'S NOTE: *Don't skip the full 30-minute wait time because it's critical for the batter to achieve proper consistency. Chickpea flour can be found at larger grocery stores, international markets, and at online markets. Top pizza crust with a thin layer of no-salt-added tomato paste, sautéed vegetables, crumbled cooked Turkey Sausage (p. 51), and thin slices of fresh mozzarella or chèvre. Broil on high for 5 minutes, until toppings are golden brown and melty. Cut into 6 slices. If you do not have a cast-iron skillet, use another oven-safe 12-inch pan, a large metal pizza pan, or a metal baking pan lined with parchment paper and well-oiled. If the latter, do not preheat, just pour the batter in. Depending on your pan's size, you may have to adjust your baking time in Step 5.*

PER SERVING: 9g protein, 9g carbohydrates, 6g fat, 1g saturated fat, 10mg sodium, 130mg potassium, 2g fiber

Rich Mushroom Gravy

Makes about 5 cups

Prep time:	20 minutes
Cooking time:	30–40 minutes
Passive time:	N/A

Budget friendly: Very

1 tablespoon dark toasted sesame oil

1 tablespoon extra-virgin olive oil

6 green onions, thinly sliced

2 shallots, minced

3 ribs celery, thinly sliced

12 ounces (350g) cremini or button mushrooms, wiped clean and thinly sliced

¼ cup (60mL) white wine (optional)

½ teaspoon freshly ground black pepper

¾ teaspoon dried sage, or 1 tablespoon minced fresh sage leaves

4 cups (.95L) Low-Sodium Vegetable Broth (p. 204), divided

3 tablespoons arrowroot powder

1 Heat the oils in a large, deep sauté pan over medium heat. Add the green onions, shallots, and celery and sauté for 8 to 10 minutes, until everything is golden. Remove the vegetables from the pan and set aside. Do not wipe out the pan; leave it on the burner.

2 Add the mushrooms to the hot pan and sauté until golden. Give them space to release their liquid so they don't get soggy.

3 Add the wine, if using, stirring to release the browned bits from the pan. If omitting the wine, substitute ¼ cup filtered water. Cook mushrooms until most of the liquid is gone.

4 Add the onion mixture back into the pan with the black pepper and sage. Sauté for 1 minute.

5 Add 3 cups of the broth. Bring to a boil.

6 In a small bowl, combine the rest of the broth with the arrowroot powder. Whisk together until smooth, then whisk in to the pot. Cook for at least 3 minutes until gravy has thickened nicely.

COOK'S NOTE: *Small mushrooms provide the best results. If you do not have arrowroot powder, substitute 2 tablespoons tapioca starch or organic cornstarch. If using the gravy for a baked filling, like a pot pie or Shepherd's pie, use one of the starches. Arrowroot does not hold its viscosity when baked. Testers added additional garlic, sage, rosemary, oregano, and chopped fresh parsley. White wine adds beautiful flavor.*

PER ¼-CUP SERVING: 2g protein, 5g carbohydrates, 1g fat, 0g saturated fat, 40mg sodium, 298mg potassium, 1g fiber

"These neuromodulation devices (Cefaly, sTMS, gammaCore, Nerivio, and Relivion) are empowering because of the absence of side effects and the liberation from the need to use medications. They are very helpful for people who want to carry on their activities of daily living, who want to manage migraine (or cluster headache with gammaCore) and not let their headaches manage them. The locus of control is with the person. You don't have to go to a doctor and get a shot or an injection or an infusion. You're not tied to me. You're liberated from me. These are really helpful options for people who want to achieve resilience, independence, and improve quality of life."

DR. STEWART TEPPER, DIRECTOR, DARTMOUTH HEADACHE CENTER

"One of the most bothersome symptoms of migraine is photophobia. If one uses Allay Lamp, a lamp that delivers a low intensity, narrow band of green light, long enough every day, it can eliminate the photophobia, reduce the intensity of the headache and the number of migraine days per month. In addition to helping during attacks, prolonged exposure to this very unique narrow band of green light can also reduce anxiety, irritability, and stress and often replace it with feelings of calm and relaxation.

In addition, users of the Allay Lamp commonly report that their sleep improved. Given that one's resilience is determined by the global wellbeing of the individual—reduced headache, anxiety, and stress— together with improved overall functioning during migraine (due to elimination of the need to seek darkness) and quality of sleep—the Allay Lamp seems a reasonable device to try."

DR. RAMI BURSTEIN, INVENTOR OF THE ALLAY LAMP, HARVARD MEDICAL SCHOOL

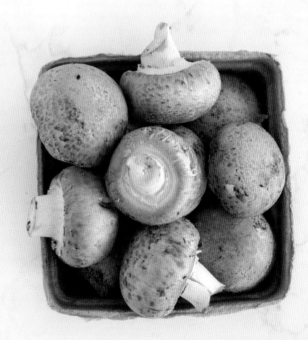

Menus for Special Occasions

Winter Holidays

Slow-Cooker Turkey Breast (p. 96) or
Roast Chicken with Veggie Gravy (p. 134)

Chipotle Sweet Potatoes (p. 112)

Green Bean Casserole (p. 116)

Mashed Potatoes (p. 117)

Rich Mushroom Gravy (p. 206)

Pumpkin Risotto (p. 121)

Stuffed Acorn Squash (p. 127)

Wild Rice Stuffing (p. 130)

Cranberry-Pear Sauce (p. 188)

Pumpkin Pie (p. 166)

Game Day

Herbed Olive Oil Crackers (p. 31) and
no-salt-added tortilla chips

Beef Barbacoa (p. 102)

Taqueria-Style Faux Guacamole (p. 189)

Mango Salsa (p. 190)

Salsa Fresca (p. 190)

Strawberry Salsa (p. 193)

Roasted Chile Pepper Hummus (p. 190,
The Migraine Relief Plan)

Salsa Verde (p. 274, *The Migraine Relief Plan*)

Sloppy Joes (p. 216, *The Migraine Relief Plan*)

Firehouse Turkey Chili (p. 213, *The
Migraine Relief Plan*)

White Chicken Chili (p. 92)

Wild Game Chili (p. 105)

Summer BBQ

Herbed Olive Oil Crackers (p. 31)

Curried Cilantro Pesto (p. 34)

Roasted Red Pepper Romesco-Style Dip (p. 32)

Curried Chicken Salad (p. 56) or Mango Chicken Salad (p. 54)

Grilled Salmon, Two Glazes (p. 65)

Mediterranean Tuna Burgers (p. 70)

Veggie Burgers (p. 71)

Blueberry Pie (p. 161)

Cherry Pie (p. 164)

Fruit Juice Gelatin (p. 181)

Grilled Peaches with Cardamom-Maple Cream Sauce (p. 256, *The Migraine Relief Plan*)

Green Salad with Bacon Salad Dressing (p. 266, *The Migraine Relief Plan*)

Lebanese Green Beans (p. 118)

Provençal Chickpea Salad (p. 218, *The Migraine Relief Plan*)

Three-Bean and Potato Salad (p. 222, *The Migraine Relief Plan*)

Berry Cobbler (p. 248, *The Migraine Relief Plan*)

Strawberry-Mint Water (p. 259, *The Migraine Relief Plan*)

Cucumber-Basil Water (p. 258, *The Migraine Relief Plan*)

Brunch

Blueberry Muffins (p. 24)

Dutch Baby Pancake (p. 49)

Eggs Benedict (p. 42)

Strata (p. 43)

Tuscan Eggs (p. 41)

Egg Mini-Quiches (p. 202, *The Migraine Relief Plan*)

Salmon-Asparagus-Thyme Omelet (p. 209, *The Migraine Relief Plan*)

Turkey Sausage Patties (p. 51)

Pork Sausage Patties (p. 208, *The Migraine Relief Plan*)

Make Your Own Bacon (p. 197, *The Migraine Relief Plan*)

Cheesecake (p. 168)

Dutch Apple Cakes (p. 169)

Strawberry-Mint Water (p. 259, *The Migraine Relief Plan*)

Cucumber-Basil Water (p. 258, *The Migraine Relief Plan*)

Resources

Blogs

KATIE GOLDEN: GoldenGraine.com

KAYLA MCCAIN: TrueKaylaisms.com

KERRIE SMYRES: TheDailyHeadache.com

JAIME MICHELE SANDERS: TheMigraineDiva.com

MICHELLE TRACY: MigraineWarriorBlog.wordpress.com

Books

10: A Memoir of Migraine Survival by Danielle Newport Fancher

Bouncing Forward: The Art and Science of Cultivating Resilience by Dr. Michaela Haas

Battle for Grace: A Memoir of Pain, Redemption, and Impossible Love by Cynthia Toussaint & John Garrett

Chronically Fabulous: Finding Wholeness and Hope Living with Chronic Illness by Marisa Zeppieri

Flying Free: My Victory Over Fear to Become the First Latina Pilot on the US Aerobatic Team by Cecilia Aragon, PhD

Gentle on My Mind: In Sickness and In Health with Glen Campbell by Kim Campbell

Love You Hard: A Memoir of Marriage, Brain Injury, and Reinventing Love by Abby Maslin

Much More Than A Headache: Understanding Migraine through Literature by Kathy O'Shea

On Being Human: A Memoir of Waking Up, Living Real, and Listening Hard by Jennifer Pastiloff

The Dizzy Cook: Managing Migraine with More Than 90 Comforting Recipes and Lifestyle Tips by Alicia Wolf

The Headache Healer's Handbook by Jan Mundo

The Migraine Relief Plan: An Eight-Week Transition to Better Eating, Fewer Headaches, and Optimal Health by Stephanie Weaver, MPH

The Part That Burns by Jeannine Ouellette

Thrive: How I Became a Superhero and *Transform to Thrive: 32 Days from Victim to Superhero* by Alexis Donkin

Through the Shadowlands: A Science Writer's Journey into an Illness Science Doesn't Understand by Julie Rehmeyer

Weed Mom: The Canna-Curious Woman's Guide to Healthier Relaxation, Happier Parenting, and Chilling TF Out by Danielle Simone Brand

Tools

ALLAY LAMP. Research-based green light therapy for migraine disease and anxiety. **AllayLamp.com**

AXON OPTICS. Migraine glasses with proprietary lenses developed by Dr. Bradley Katz at the University of Utah. **AxonOptics.com**

CEFALY. Over-the-counter neuromodulation device to treat and prevent migraine attacks. **Cefaly.com**

SPOONK. Acupressure mats for deep relaxation. **SpoonkSpace.com**

THERASPECS. Fashionable and therapeutic blue light glasses for light sensitivity, migraine, and post-concussion relief. **TheraSpecs.com**

THUMPER. Percussive massagers. **ThumperMassager.com**

Websites

AMERICAN HEADACHE SOCIETY. A professional society of headache doctors and researchers providing scientific resources for healthcare professionals; helpful for patients who want to educate themselves on the latest studies. **AmericanHeadacheSociety.org**

AMERICAN MIGRAINE FOUNDATION. Patient support and advocacy as well as driving research. Resource library and patient guides. **AmericanMigraineFoundation.org**

ASSOCIATION OF MIGRAINE DISORDERS. Healthcare provider resources, the Spotlight on Migraine podcast, as well as the Shades for Migraine advocacy day. **MigraineDisorders.org**

DAWN C. BUSE, PHD. Dawn Buse is a psychologist at the Albert Einstein College of Medicine. Her site provides many free guided meditations. **www.DawnBuse.com**

CHRONIC MIGRAINE AWARENESS, INC. Advocacy and awareness campaigns, including triage kits, merchandise, and downloadable graphics. **ChronicMigraineAwareness.org**

CLUSTERBUSTERS. Raising awareness and educating physicians about cluster headache, supporting enrollment in clinical trials, and raising money for research. **Clusterbusters.org**

CLUSTER HEADACHE SUPPORT GROUP. Community and educational resources for people living with cluster headache. **chsg.org**

> "Just know that in the darkest of times the sun rises again, and we will be better for our struggles and have more knowledge."
>
> DR. SUSAN MATHISON, FOUNDER, CATALYST MEDICAL CENTER AND SPA

COALITION FOR HEADACHE AND MIGRAINE PATIENTS (CHAMP). CHAMP brings together the most influential patient advocacy organizations and leaders in the area of migraine, cluster, and headache diseases to more effectively fight stigma and help people achieve fair access to treatments. **HeadacheMigraine.org**

CREATING RESILIENCE. Personal coaching with mindfulness-based stress reduction to build resilience with Margot Anderson. **Creating-Resilience.com**

DANIELLE BYRON HENRY MIGRAINE FOUNDATION. Its mission is to increase access to care, especially for young adults and children, by educating primary care providers in the treatment of migraine. **DanielleFoundation.org**

DANIELLE HECK, MS, OTR/L, OCCUPATIONAL THERAPIST. Helps people learn to manage migraine, identify triggers, and develop healthy habits so they can take back control of their lives. **MigraineTherapist.com**

FOR GRACE. To increase awareness and promote education of the gender disparity women experience in the assessment and treatment of their pain. **ForGrace.org**

HEADACHE AND MIGRAINE POLICY FORUM. Advances public policies and practices that promote accelerated innovation and improved treatments for persons living with headache and migraine disease. **HeadacheMigraineForum.org**

HEALTHYWOMEN. The leading independent, nonprofit health information source for women in the U.S. **Healthywomen.org**

HOPE FOR MIGRAINE COMMUNITY. A supportive group for people with migraine who are taking or interested in CGRP medications. **MigraineMeanderings.com**

LINDSAY WEITZEL, PHD. Lindsay works with those who have chronic migraine to help them build a rock wall of strategies to manage their migraine disease; half the wall is medications, half is their life factors, the mortar is their mentality. **LindsayWeitzel.com**

LUPUS FOUNDATION OF AMERICA. Advocacy to generate support for people affected by lupus. **Lupus.org**

MIGRAINE. A for-profit website for migraine patients operated by Health Central. Features top migraine bloggers, an annual reader survey, and many patient information resources. **Migraine.com**

MIGRAINE AGAIN. A collection of website articles, newsletters, videos, podcasts, interviews, and resources. **MigraineAgain.com**

MIGRAINEDISEASE.ORG. The only patient-owned and -operated migraine website that medically reviews all content. **MigraineDisease.org**

MIGRAINE RELIEF RECIPES. Over 400 whole-foods recipes, many of them adapted to fit the Plan. **MigraineReliefRecipes.com**

MIGRAINE WORLD SUMMIT. The largest virtual patient event in the world for those with chronic headache and migraine disease. Previous episodes available year-round (paywall); annual event is free while live. **MigraineWorldSummit.com**

MILES FOR MIGRAINE. Creates community at fun walk/run events, educational programs, and support groups while raising money for migraine research. **MilesForMigraine.org**

NATIONAL HEADACHE FOUNDATION. Provides educational resources for patients and caregivers. **Headaches.org**

PATIENT ADVOCATE FOUNDATION. Provides educational materials that help patients self-advocate to overcome common challenges. **PatientAdvocate.org**

THE MIGRAINE DIETITIAN, KELLI YATES, RDN, LD, CLT. Kelli is a functional dietitian specializing in the role of gut health and hormones in migraine management. **KelliYatesNutrition.com**

U.S. PAIN FOUNDATION. Empowers, educates, connects, and advocates for individuals living with chronic illness that causes pain, as well as their caregivers and clinicians. **USPainFoundation.org**

VESTIBULAR DISORDERS ASSOCIATION. Provides educational and support resources to people with inner ear and brain balance disorders, including migraine-associated vertigo. **Vestibular.org**

Acknowledgments

To my wonderful recipe testers: Saadia Ali Esmail, Barb Anderson, Julie Botes, Heather Collins, Anne Fetsko, Katrina Fox, Dafne Gokcen, Christine Gurrera, Eugenia Hall, Azlynn Hare, Louise Helcoop, Gwen Hughes, Daisy Jeys, Kerry Johnson, Jason Klassen, Andrea Larkin, Kristi Mai, Camilla M. Mann, Noelle McClure, Tricia Mihal, Wilma Myers, Marcus C. Simpson, Lexie Smith-Kliebe, Erica N. Timmerman, Valerie Willardson.

To my neighbors, who are always willing to loan pans, ingredients, and taste-test: Amanda, Ashley, Bonnie, Katie, Sharon, Tori.

To my agent Sally Ekus, my photographer Laura Bashar, and the team at Agate Publishing: Doug Seibold, Jane Seibold, Jacqueline Jarik, book designer Morgan Krehbiel, and editors Amanda Gibson, Naomi Huffman, and Liza Schoenfein.

To my contributors and encouragers: Margot Anderson, Cecilia Aragon, PhD, Anita L. Arambula, Danielle Simone Brand, Eileen Brewer, Rami Burstein, MD, Dawn Buse, PhD, Kim Campbell, Alexis Donkin, Paula Dumas, Maddy Dychtwald, Madushree Ghosh, Katie Golden, Melissa Gould, Mahshid Fashandi Hager, Michaela Haas, PhD, Ricki Heller, Wendy Holloway, Cynthia James, Kimberly Joy, Shirley Kessel, Domenica Marchetti, Abby Maslin, Susan Mathison, MD, Kayla McCain, Nancie McDermott, Kathy O'Shea, Jeannine Ouellette, Jennifer Pastiloff, Julie Rehmeyer, Jennifer Robblee, MD, Jaime Michele Sanders, Elizabeth Seng, PhD, Hart Shafer, Margaret Slavin, PhD, RDN, Kerrie Smyres, Stewart Tepper, MD, Cynthia Toussaint, Lindsay Burgello Weitzel, PhD, Kelli Yates, RDN, CLT, Marisa Zeppieri.

And to Microwave Boy, who has eaten every bite.

Thank you all.

Endnotes

1   GBD 2016 Disease and Injury Incidence and Prevalence Collaborators. 'Global, regional, and national incidence, prevalence, and years lived with disability for 328 diseases and injuries for 195 countries, 1990-2016: a systematic analysis for the Global Burden of Disease Study 2016,' The Lancet, 390, no. 10100, (2017 Sep 16):1211-1259.

2   Lipton, R.B., Serrano, D., Holland, S., Fanning K.M., Reed, M.L., Buse, D.C. 'Barriers to the diagnosis and treatment of migraine: effects of sex, income, and headache features,' Headache, 53, no. 1 (Jan 2013): 81-92.

3   Lipton, R.B., Buse, D.C., Serrano, D., Holland, S., Reed, M.L. 'Examination of unmet treatment needs among persons with episodic migraine: results of the American Migraine Prevalence and Prevention (AMPP) Study,' Headache, 53, no. 8, (Sep 2013):1300-11.

4   Haut, S.R., Bigal, M.E., Lipton, R.B. 'Chronic disorders with episodic manifestations: focus on epilepsy and migraine,' The Lancet Neurology, 5, no. 2, (Feb 2006):148-157.

5   Hébert, J.R., Shivappa, N., Wirth, M.D., Hussey, J.R., Hurley, T.G. 'Perspective: The Dietary Inflammatory Index (DII)—Lessons Learned, Improvements Made, and Future Directions,' Advances in Nutrition, 10, no. 2, (2019):185-195.

6   Phillips, C.M., Chen, L.-W., Heude, B., Bernard, J.Y., Harvey, N.C., Duijts, L., Mensink-Bout, S.M., Polanska, K., Mancano, G., Suderman, M., Shivappa, N., Hébert, J.R. 'Dietary Inflammatory Index and Non-Communicable Disease Risk: A Narrative Review,' Nutrients, 11, no. 8, (2019):1873.

7   Ramsden, C.E., Zamora, D., Faurot, K.R., MacIntosh, B., Horowitz, M., Keyes, G.S., Yuan, Z.-X., Miller, V., Lynch, C., Honvoh, G., Park, J., Levy, R., Domenichiello, A.F., Johnston, A., Majchrzak-Hong, S., Hibbeln, J.R., Barrow, D.A., Loewke, J., Davis, J.M., Mannes, A., Palsson, O.S., Suchindran, C.M., Gaylord, S.A., Mann, J.D., 'Dietary alteration of n-3 and n-6 fatty acids for headache reduction in adults with migraine: randomized controlled trial,' British Medical Journal. Published online June 30, 2021:n1448.

8   Pérez-Muñoz, A., Buse, D.C., Andrasik, F. 'Behavioral Interventions for Migraine,' Neurologic Clinics, 37, no. 4, (Nov 2019):789-813.

9   Ramsden, CE, Zamora, D, Faurot, KR, MacIntosh, B, Horowitz, M, Keyes, GS, Yuan, Z-X, Miller, V, Lynch, C, Honvoh, G, Park, J, Levy, R, Domenichiello, AF, Johnston, A, Majchrzak-Hong, S, Hibbeln, JR, Barrow, DA, Loewke, J, Davis, JM, Mannes, A, Palsson, OS, Suchindran, CM, Gaylord, SA, Mann, JD, 'Dietary alteration of n-3 and n-6 fatty acids for headache reduction in adults with migraine: randomized controlled trial,' British Medical Journal. Published online June 30, 2021:n1448.

10 Buse, D.C., Rupnow, M.F.T., Lipton R.B, 'Assessing and managing all aspects of migraine: Migraine attacks, migraine-related functional impairment, common comorbidities, and quality of life,' Mayo Clinic Proceedings, 84 (2009):422-435.

Recipe Index

Recipe	Vegan/Vegetarian	Dairy-Free	Egg-Free	Grain-Free
Snacks				
Trail Mix	V	DF	EF	GF
Chewy Cherry Oat Bars	V	DF		
Blueberry Muffins	V	DF		
Shamrock Smoothie	V	DF	EF	GF
Creamy Not-ella Carob Butter	V	DF	EF	GF
Herbed Olive Oil Crackers	V	DF	EF	
Roasted Red Pepper Romesco-Style Dip	V	DF	EF	GF
Curried Cilantro Pesto	V	DF	EF	GF
Breakfast				
Breakfast Hash	V	DF	EF	GF
Quickie Microwave Egg Scramble	V			GF
Tuscan Eggs	V	DF		GF
Eggs Benedict	V			
Strata	V	DF		
Pumpkin-Spice Waffles	V	DF	EF	
Dutch Baby Pancake	V	DF		GF
Tex-Mex Migas	V	DF		
Turkey Sausage Patties		DF	EF	GF
Salads and Light Meals				
Mango Chicken Salad		DF	EF	GF
Curried Chicken Salad		DF	EF	GF
Grilled Chicken Caesar Salad		DF	EF	GF
Fattoush Salad	V	DF	EF	GF
Tuna-Rice Salad		DF	EF	
Honey-Mustard Salmon Salad		DF	EF	GF
Grilled Salmon, Two Glazes		DF	EF	GF
Quinrizo Taco Salad	V	DF	EF	

Recipe	Vegan/ Vegetarian	Dairy-Free	Egg-Free	Grain-Free
Quick and Easy Ramen	V	DF	EF	
Mediterranean Tuna Burgers		DF	EF	GF
Veggie Burgers	V	DF	EF	
Weekend Meals				
Carrot-Ginger Soup	V	DF	EF	GF
Creamy Potato Soup	V	DF	EF	GF
Detox Veggie Soup	V	DF	EF	GF
Gazpacho	V	DF	EF	
Parsnip-Leek Soup	V	DF	EF	GF
Spicy Sweet Potato Soup	V	DF	EF	GF
Twice-Baked Thai-Spiced Potatoes	V	DF	EF	GF
South Asian-Inspired Chickpea Masala	V	DF	EF	GF
Spicy Black Bean and Rice Casserole	V			
Sheet Pan Chicken Thighs		DF	EF	GF
Lazy Chicken and Broth		DF	EF	GF
Cozy Chicken and Rice		DF	EF	
White Chicken Chili		DF	EF	GF
Turkey Mole Tamale Pie		DF	EF	
Slow-Cooker Turkey Breast		DF	EF	GF
Quick Turkey Tacos		DF	EF	
Super-Simple Beef Stew		DF	EF	GF
Beef Barbacoa		DF	EF	GF
Wild Game Chili		DF	EF	GF
Chili-Mac Skillet Dinner		DF	EF	
Scrumptious Sides				
Coconut-Curried Greens	V	DF	EF	GF
Chipotle Sweet Potatoes	V		EF	GF
Sweet Potato Oven Fries	V	DF	EF	GF
Curried Roast Cauliflower	V	DF	EF	GF
Green Bean Casserole	V	DF	EF	
Garlic Mashed Potatoes	V	DF	EF	GF
Lebanese Green Beans	V	DF	EF	GF

Recipe	Vegan/ Vegetarian	Dairy-Free	Egg-Free	Grain-Free
Saffron Rice	V	DF	EF	
Pumpkin Risotto	V	DF	EF	
Ratatouille	V	DF	EF	GF
Roasted Garlic-Jalapeño Grits	V	DF	EF	
Oven-Roasted Vegetables with Greek Spice Blend	V	DF	EF	GF
Stuffed Acorn Squash	V	DF	EF	
Pan-Roasted Kale with Crispy Italian Breadcrumbs	V	DF	EF	
Wild Rice Stuffing	V	DF	EF	
Progressive Cooking				
Roasted Chicken with Veggie Gravy		DF	EF	
Low-Sodium Chicken Broth		DF	EF	GF
Perfect Chicken Soup		DF	EF	GF
Thai-Style Chicken Soup		DF	EF	
Beany-Brothy Deliciousness	V	DF	EF	GF
Puréed Vegetable Soup	V	DF	EF	GF
Tuscan White Bean Soup	V	DF	EF	GF
Pasta e Fagioli	V	DF	EF	
Quick Bean Tacos	V	DF	EF	
Easy Roasted Potatoes	V	DF	EF	GF
Cauliflower-Chickpea Curry	V	DF	EF	GF
Thai-Style Shrimp Curry		DF	EF	GF
Potato Cakes	V	DF		
Tex-Mex Skillet Dinner		DF	EF	GF
Desserts				
Blueberry Pie	V		EF	
Gluten-Free Pastry Crust	V		EF	
Cherry Pie	V		EF	
Peach Crumble Pie	V		EF	
Pumpkin Pie	V	DF		GF
Apple-Spice Mug Cake	V	DF		
Cheesecake	V			GF

Recipe	Vegan/Vegetarian	Dairy-Free	Egg-Free	Grain-Free
Dutch Apple Cake	V	DF		
Birthday Cake with Fudgy Frosting	V	DF		
Tapioca Pudding	V	DF		GF
Strawberry Sorbet	V	DF	EF	GF
Choco-Berry Sorbet	V	DF	EF	GF
Sunbutter Freezer Fudge	V	DF	EF	GF
Fruit Juice Gelatin		DF	EF	GF
Sauces, Condiments, and Basics				
Cherry-Sesame Dressing	V	DF	EF	GF
Mango-Jalapeño Dressing	V	DF	EF	GF
Shallot-Mustard Vinaigrette	V	DF	EF	GF
Chunky Tomato Sauce	V	DF	EF	GF
Cranberry-Pear Sauce	V	DF	EF	GF
Taqueria-Style Faux Guacamole	V	DF	EF	GF
Mango Salsa	V	DF	EF	GF
Salsa Fresca	V	DF	EF	GF
Strawberry Salsa	V	DF	EF	GF
Egg-Free Mayonnaise	V	DF	EF	GF
Olive Oil Mayonnaise	V	DF		GF
Hot Sauce	V	DF	EF	GF
Ketchup	V	DF	EF	GF
Thai Curry Paste (Green and Red)	V	DF	EF	GF
Garam Masala	V	DF	EF	GF
Greek Spice Blend	V	DF	EF	GF
Pumpkin Pie Spice	V	DF	EF	GF
Seafood Seasoning	V	DF	EF	GF
Spice Rub for Red Meat	V	DF	EF	GF
Taco Seasoning	V	DF	EF	GF
Gluten-Free Flour Blend	V	DF	EF	
Low-Sodium Vegetable Broth	V	DF	EF	GF
Quick Pizza Crust	V	DF	EF	GF
Rich Mushroom Gravy	V	DF	EF	GF

Index